Highlights in Gastrointestinal Oncology

FALK SYMPOSIUM 149

Highlights in Gastrointestinal Oncology

Edited by

E. van Cutsem
University Hospital
Leuven
Belgium

A.K. Rustgi
University of Pennsylvania
Philadelphia, PA
USA

W. Schmiegel
Ruhr University
Bochum
Germany

M. Zeitz
Charité Medical University
Berlin
Germany

Proceedings of the Falk Symposium 149 held in Berlin, Germany,
October 1–2, 2005

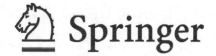 Springer

Library of Congress Cataloging-in-Publication Data is available.

ISBN-10 1-4020-5108-5
ISBN-13 978-1-4020-5108-1

Published by Springer,
PO Box 17, 3300 AA Dordrecht, The Netherlands

Sold and distributed in North, Central and South America
by Springer,
101 Philip Drive, Norwell, MA 02061 USA

In all other countries, sold and distributed
by Springer,
PO Box 322, 3300 AH Dordrecht, The Netherlands

Printed on acid-free paper

Printed and bound in Great Britain by MPG Books Limited, Bodmin, Cornwall.

Contents

List of principal contributors

H-P Allgaier
Innere Medizin
HELIOS Klinik
Jostalstr. 12
D-79822 Titisee-Neustadt
Germany

L Attisano
Department of Biochemistry
Terrance Donnelly Centre for
  Cellular and Biomolecular
  Research, Room 1008
160 College Street,
University of Toronto
Toronto, Ontario, M5S 3E1
Canada

J Behrens
Nikolaus-Fiebiger Centre for
  Molecular Medicine
University of Erlangen-Nuremberg
Glückstr. 6
D-91054 Erlangen
Germany

M Bissonnette
University of Chicago
Department of Medicine
Section of Gastroenterology
MC 4076
5841 S. Maryland Avenue
Chicago, IL 60615
USA

W Fischbach
Medizinische Klinik II
Klinikum Aschaffenburg
Am Hasenkopf
D-63739 Aschaffenburg
Germany

JR Jass
Department of Pathology
McGill University
Duff Medical Building
3775 University Street
Montreal, Quebec
Canada

A Jung
Pathologisches Institut der Ludwig-
  Maximilians Universität München
Thalkirchner Str. 36
D-80337 München
Germany

D Lieberman
Division of Gastroenterology
Oregon Health Sciences University
Portland VA Medical Center P3-GI
PO Box 1034
Portland, OR 97239
USA

MF Neurath
Laboratory of Immunology
I. Department of Medicine
University of Mainz
Langenbeckstrasse 1
D-55131 Mainz
Germany

S Petrasch
Innere Medizin
Klinikum Duisburg
Wedau-Kliniken
Zu den Rehwiesen 9
D-47055 Duisburg
Germany

C Rödel
Klinik für Strahlentherapie
Universität Erlangen
Universitätsstrasse 27
D-91054 Erlangen
Germany

JR Siewert
Klinikum rechts der Isar der
    Technische Universität
Chirurgie
Ismaninger Str. 22
D-81675 München
Germany

MM Taketo
Kyoto University School of Medicine
Department of Pharmacology
54 Shogoin, Kawahara-cho
Sakyo-ku
Kyoto 606 8043
Japan

Y Wang
Veridex, LLC, a Johnson and
    Johnson Company
3210 Merryfield Row
San Diego, CA 92121
USA

SJ Winawer
Gastroenterology and Nutrition
    Service
Memorial Sloan-Kettering Cancer
    Center
1275 York Avenue, Box 90
New York, NY 10021
USA

AG Zauber
Memorial Sloan-Ketting Cancer
    Center
Department of Epidemiology and
    Biostatistics
1275 York Avenue
New York, NY 10021
USA

W Zhou
Deparment of Hematology and
    Oncology
The Winship Cancer Institute of
    Emory University
Building C, Room 4084
1365 Clifton Road, NE
Atlanta, GA 30322
USA

List of chairpersons

R Arnold
Innere Medizin
Klinikum der Universität
Baldingerstr.
D-35043 Marburg
Germany

J Behrens
Nikolaus-Fiebiger Centre for
  Molecular Medicine
University of Erlangen-Nuremberg
Glückstr. 6
D-91054 Erlangen
Germany

M Classen
Innere Medizin II
Klinikum rechts der Isar der
  Technischen Universität
Ismaninger Str. 22
D-81675 München
Germany

E van Cutsem
Univ. Ziekenhuis Gasthuisberg
Department of Gastroenterology
Herestraat 49
B-3000 Leuven
Belgium

R DuBois
Vanderbilt University
School of Medicine
Department of Gastroenterology
21st Avenue, South at Garland
  Avenue
Nashville, TN 37232
USA

W Fischbach
Medizinische Klinik II
Klinikum Aschaffenburg
Am Hasenkopf
D-63739 Aschaffenburg
Germany

U Graeven
Innere Medizin I
Krankenhaus St. Franziskus
Viersener Str. 450
D-41063 Mönchengladbach
Germany

S Hahn
Medizin Universitäts-Klinik
Knappschaftskrankenhaus
In der Schornau 23–25
D-44892 Bochum
Germany

M Heike
Innere Medizin – Gastroenterologie
Klinikzentrum Mitte
Klinikum Dortmund
Beurhausstr. 40
D-44137 Dortmund
Germany

W Hohenberger
Chirurgie
Universität Erlangen-Nürnberg
Krankenhausstr. 12
D-91054 Erlangen
Germany

HI Hurwitz
Duke University Medical Center
Department of Medical Oncology
  and Transplantation
Box 3052
PO Box 17969
Durham, NC 27710
USA

M von Knebel Doeberitz
Pathologie
Klinikum der Universität
Im Neuenheimer Feld 220/221
D-69120 Heidelberg
Germany

MM Lerch
Gastroenterologie, Endokrinologie
  und Ernährungsmedizin
Universitätsklinikum Greifswald der
  Ernst-Moritz-Arndt-Universität
  Greifswald
Friedrich-Loeffler-Str. 23a
D-17487 Greifswald
Germany

C Louvet
Hôpital Saint-Antoine
Service d'Oncologie
184 rue du Faubourg St. Antoine
F-75571 Paris
France

P Propping
Humangenetik
Universitätsklinikum Bonn
Wilhelmstr. 31
D-53111 Bonn
Germany

R Reinacher-Schick
Medizinische Universitätsklinik
Knappschaftskrankenhaus
In der Schornau 23–25
D-44892 Bochum
Germany

G Trenn
Innere Medizin
Knappschaftskrankenhaus
Osterfelder Str. 157
D-46242 Bottrop
Germany

M Zeitz
Innere Medizin I
Charité Universitätsmedizin
Campus Benjamin Franklin (CBF)
Hindenburgdamm 30
D-12203 Berlin
Germany

Preface

Cancers of the digestive tract account for a large portion of all malignancies and colorectal cancer (CRC), the most common digestive tract cancer, is the second leading cause of cancer death in the Western World. Although a number of advances have been made in understanding the pathogenesis of the diseases and in developing new treatments in particular for CRC patients the mortality of GI cancers is still considerably high. Recent trends in medical and surgical oncology, gastroenterology and molecular pathology are of considerable interest in dealing with this problem. New models for the carcinogenesis of esophageal cancer have been developed potentially leading to new chemopreventive strategies for the disease, *Helicobacter pylori* has been identified as the leading cause of gastric lymphomatous as well as epithelial malignancies, alternative molecular pathways of colon cancer development have been identified and above all novel treatments have been found which target specific molecular alterations of malignant cells and thus significantly improve overall survival of GI cancer patients.

This conference was dedicated to a comprehensive overview of the recent advances in GI Oncology. The outstanding contribution of world leading experts in the various fields has achieved an up-to-date analysis of the scientific data also providing immediate applications for day-to-day clinical work. The conference has also expressed the hope that through a better understanding of the molecular alterations which lead to GI cancers partly through using sophisticated new laboratory techniques we will be able to identify novel targets for prevention and treatment of the diseases. Among the various highlights of the conference were lectures on animal models for GI cancers, on statistical models to compute polyp recurrence after polypectomies, concepts to improve public awareness for GI cancers as well as basic science concepts about to enter clinical use.

The organizers appreciate the time and effort of each individual author. We also would like to thank all the numerous people who helped us organize this symposium. In particular, we would like to thank Dr. M. Falk who gave the necessary financial support and Mrs. S. Maresch, Freiburg as well as Ms. G. Rohe, Bochum who were of great help in organizing this meeting.

A. Reinacher-Schick and W. Schmiegel
on behalf of the Scientific Organizers
E. Van Cutsem, Leuven, A.K. Rustgi, Philadelphia,
W. Schmiegel, Bochum and M. Zeitz, Berlin

Section I
Oesophageal cancer: aetiology, screening and treatment

Chair: W. FISCHBACH and M. HEIKE

1
State-of-the-Art Lecture:
Of mice and men: mouse models for colon carcinogenesis

M. M. TAKETO

INTRODUCTION

Mortality in colon cancer takes one of the highest positions among all cancer deaths in many countries. As opposed to lung cancer, the majority of which cases should be prevented by elimination of tobacco smoke, there is no established environmental factor that can help eliminate colon cancer formation. To establish therapeutic and preventive strategies, it would be very important to develop workable mouse models. Based on its genetic origin, colon cancer can be divided into two classes: polyposis colon cancer and non-polyposis colon cancer. Many genes whose mutations are responsible for colon carcinogenesis have been discovered through molecular genetic studies of hereditary cancer predisposition syndromes such as familial adenomatous polyposis (FAP), and hereditary non-polyposis colon cancer (HNPCC). Induced mutations in mice of these genes have provided mouse models that are similar to human colon cancer and polyposis, even though they may not be identical to the human diseases. These mouse models have provided a large body of experimental evidence that helps us to understand the initiation, expansion and progression of colon tumorigenesis. These model mice have also turned out to be very useful tools to test chemotherapeutic and preventive agents. Here I will review recent progress in the field with some emphasis on the work from my own laboratory.

MOUSE MODELS FOR FAP

FAP is a hereditary disease with dominant inheritance that causes numerous colon polyps. Although the polyps consist of benign adenomas, some of them will develop into malignant adenocarcinomas eventually, if left untreated. The adenomatous polyposis coli (APC) gene was identified on 5q as one of the genes commonly deleted in some FAP kindreds[1,2]. It encodes a huge protein of about

3

2850 amino acid residues, forms a complex with axin and helps glycogen synthase kinase (GSK) 3β to phosphorylate N-terminal serine/threonine residues of β-catenin, accelerating its rapid degradation through ubiquitination[3]. If the *APC* gene is mutated, GSK3β cannot phosphorylate β-catenin. Unphosphorylated and therefore stabilized β-catenin accumulates in the cytoplasm, moves to the nucleus where it activates TCF/LEF transcription factors, inducing a set of new genes; Wnt target genes[4]. Activation of the Wnt pathway in the colonic epithelium appears to be one of the key events in the polyp initiation process[5].

Apc[Min] mice, *Apc*[Δ716] mice, *Apc*[1638N] mice and other *Apc* mutant mice

The first mouse mutant in the *Apc* gene (the mouse homologue of human *APC* on mouse Chr 18) was discovered from a colony of randomly mutagenized mice[6]. This mutant, *Min* (multiple intestinal neoplasia) was found to carry a truncation mutation at codon 850 of the *Apc* gene[7], hence *Apc*[Min]. In the C57BL/6 background the heterozygote develops ~30 polyps in the small intestine. With gene knockout technology several *Apc* mutations have been constructed. *Apc*[Δ716] contains truncating mutation at codon 716, whereas *Apc*[1638N] does so at codon 1638[8,9]. As in *Apc*[Min] mice, both knockout mutants develop polyps mainly in the small intestine. Histologically, all these *Apc* mutants form polyp adenomas indistinguishable from each other. Interestingly, however, the polyp numbers are very different, even in the same C57BL/6J background. Namely, *Apc*[Δ716] develops usually ~300 polyps, whereas *Apc*[1638N] forms only ~3 polyps. Despite the numerous polyps developing in the small intestine in the *Apc*[Δ716] (as well as in *Apc*[Min]) mice, only a few polyps are formed in the colon, although the penetrance is complete. Because this polyp localization phenotype is just opposite to that in human FAP, in which the polyps are formed mostly in the colon, and very rarely in the small intestine, it has been questioned whether *Apc* mutant mice can be accurate models for human FAP. We have recently constructed a mutant mouse strain in which numerous polyps develop in the distal colon[10]. Using *Apc*[Δ716] mice it was demonstrated that polyp formation is initiated by loss of heterozygosity (LOH) at the *Apc* locus in the proliferative zone cells[9], followed by formation of an outpocket in the intestinal crypt[5]. The results strongly suggested that APC protein is essential for the proliferative zone cells to migrate along the crypt–villus axis, which is consistent with additional pieces of recent circumstantial evidence. Although aberrant crypt foci (ACF) have been proposed to be the precursor of the polyps in humans as well as in rodents, the term does not represent a histopathological entity. Azoxymethane-treated rat colon contains two types of microscopic lesions, and the one with β-catenin mutation and nuclear accumulation does not resemble ACF[11]. These microadenomas, lacking the appearance of ACF, are likely to be the precursors of colon cancer[12].

Several other *Apc* gene knockout mice have been reported. Their histopathology appears essentially the same as in *Apc*[Min] or *Apc*[Δ716], with the only difference being the number of the intestinal polyps.

Modifier genes of *Apc* intestinal polyposis

When Apc^{Min} mutation is transferred to AKR mice, the intestinal polyp number decreases to only 1–3, due to a modifying locus *Mom* (modifier of Min)-*1* on Chr 4^{13}. Based on the results of a genetic analysis, this modifier was proposed to encode a secretory form of phospholipase A_2 (sPLA$_2$), but further analysis revealed a cluster of several secretory phospholipases in the locus[14]. Because sPLA$_2$ cleaves long-chain fatty acids from membrane phospholipids, it is difficult to explain the *Mom-1* phenotype by the enzyme activity. Namely, sPLA$_2$ is wild-type in AKR, and mutated in C57BL/6. Thus, one would expect that an increased amount of arachidoic acid (AA) is released and supplied to cyclooxygenases (COX) that produce tumour-promoting prostaglandins in the wild-type, which should lead to higher numbers of intestinal polyps in AKR; just the opposite phenotype from the experimental results above. In addition to *Mom-1*, the mouse strain CAST carries a dominant modifier gene that confers significant protection against Apc^{Min} intestinal polyposis, although the gene remains to be identified and characterized[14].

Introduction of COX-2 gene mutation dramatically decreases the polyp number in *Apc* polyposis mice[15,16]. Likewise, COX-1 mutation also reduces the polyp multiplicity in *Apc* polyposis mice.

We first determined expression of COX-2 protein in intestinal polyps of various sizes, and found that COX-2 was expressed from a very early stage of polyp formation[17]. We then introduced a COX-2 gene (*Ptgs2*) knockout mutation into the $Apc^{\Delta716}$ mice, and discovered that both the number and size of polyps were reduced dramatically in the compound mutant mice, in a mutated gene dosage-dependent manner. To confirm the results with pharmaceutical compounds, we further dosed $Apc^{\Delta716}$ mice with COX-2 inhibitors, and demonstrated that the polyp number can be reduced in a dosage-dependent manner[17,18]. These results gave the rationale to treat human FAP patients with COX-2 inhibitors such as celecoxib or rofecoxib, and clinical trials confirmed the results of animal experiments[19]. Following these experiments, a number of reports have been published describing dosing *Apc* mutant mice with various drugs or drug candidates. We have summarized such experiments in a recent review[20]. It should be noted that the constitutive isozyme COX-1 also plays a significant role in polyposis. Introduction of COX-1 mutation into Apc^{Min} mice reduces the number and size of intestinal polyps by $\sim 80\%$, a similar effect by COX-2 mutation[21]. COX-1 and COX-2 cooperate in polyp formation by supplying prostaglandin PGE$_2$ that stimulates polyp angiogenesis[22]. These results can explain why aspirin reduces colon cancer incidence despite the fact that it is essentially a COX-1 inhibitor.

To assess the role of the AA/COX-2/PGE$_2$ pathway further, we constructed several additional compound mutants of $Apc^{\Delta716}$ mice with other genes in the pathway. Although cyclooxygenase is the rate-limiting enzyme in the pathway, its substrate AA is not freely available *in vivo*, but supplied on demand by the activity of phospholipases that cleaves AA from membrane phospholipids. One of the key enzymes in this activity is cytosolic phospholipase A_2 (cPLA$_2$). We introduced a knockout gene for the enzyme into $Apc^{\Delta716}$ mice, and demonstrated that polyp expansion is reduced significantly[23]. In the

5

downstream of the pathway, on the other hand, the direct metabolite of AA by COX is PGH_2 that is converted further to various prostanoids as such as PGA_2, D_2, $F_{2\alpha}$, E_2, I_2, and thromboxane A_2 (TXA_2). Among them PGE_2 appears to play the major role in polyposis by binding to four G-protein-coupled cell surface receptors, EP1, EP2, EP3 and/or EP4. To determine which particular EP receptor is involved in the polyposis phenotype, we introduced knockout mutations for the receptors into $Apc^{\Delta716}$ mice, respectively, and scored the polyp number and size. The results clearly showed a significant suppression of the polyposis phenotype only in the compound mutant mice with EP2 mutation[24]. Moreover, we found that induction of COX-2 itself, as well as other phenotypes associated with COX-2 induction such as angiogenesis and basement membrane changes, are also mediated by PGE_2 and EP2 receptor. The former phenotype indicates that a positive feedback signal mediated through EP2 and intracellular cyclic AMP regulates COX-2 expression[24].

Expression of COX-2 has been observed not only in adenomatous polyps, but also in hamartomatous polyps and malignant cancers. For example, COX-2 expression has been reported in Peutz–Jeghers gastrointestinal hamartomas[25]. We have recently investigated expression of COX-2 in hamartomas of three models, namely, in mutant mice of *Smad4*, *Cdx2* and *Lkb1*, and found significant expression levels in all models[26]. These results indicate that COX-2 induction is a general phenomenon common to most tumours.

While other possible targets have been proposed for the antitumour activities of non-steroidal anti-inflammatory drugs (NSAID)[27], these pathways remain to be investigated further by genetic means, i.e. crossing of the target gene knockout mice with the polyposis mice.

Another avenue of similar experiments is to study the effects of various diets and food additives, in attempts to identify the epidemiological effects on cancer initiation and progression. For example, we demonstrated that docosahexaenoic acid (DHA) reduces intestinal polyp development, although the effect is moderate and found only in female mice[28], whereas feeding $Apc^{\Delta716}$ mice with high-fat diet increases polyp numbers significantly[29]. Likewise, a Western-style diet (high fat and low calcium) accelerates tumour formation in Apc^{1638N} mice[30]. It is also interesting to point out that calorie intake restriction by 40% reduces intestinal polyps in Apc^{Min} mice by $\sim60\%$, suggesting that dietary interventions can partially offset genetic susceptibility to intestinal carcinogenesis[31].

As described above, all *Apc* mutant mice develop adenomatous polyps in the small intestine, rather than in the colon. However, recent studies show that an additional mutation in the *Cdx2* gene in $Apc^{\Delta716}$ mice reverses the polyp localization, shifting most polyps to the colon as in human FAP[10]. Interestingly, the dramatic increase in colon polyp number is caused by the increased frequency of *Apc* LOH caused by chromosomal instability. The latter results from activation of the mTOR pathway and acceleration of the G_1 to S phase transition in the cell cycle[10]. These results present a new mechanism for chromosomal instability, and suggest a possibility of treatment and prevention of colon cancer with chromosomal instability.

Mutations in DNA mismatch repair genes

Mutations in DNA mismatch repair genes are involved in HNPCC, and show microsatellite instability (MSI), a mutator phenotype[32,33]. The proteins involved in DNA mismatch repair consist of three classes: those essential for cell viability (MSH2 and MLH1), non-essential redundant genes (MSH3 and 6, PMS1, MLH3, and EXO1), and genes also involved in essential DNA replication processes (PCNA, RFC, RPA, DNA polymerase δ)[34]. Although knockout mutations have been introduced to many of these genes in the mouse, most intestinal tumours in these mice are adenomas, and malignant adenocarcinomas are very rare. Accordingly, these mice with single gene mutations are not practical models for colon cancer; rather they are more suitable for analysis of early changes in the DNA mismatch repair lesions. Interestingly, however, compound mutants of these genes are more severe in their phenotypes, and some develop adenocarcinomas, although none of them are metastatic (see below).

Homozygous mutant mice in *Msh6*, one of the genes involved in DNA mismatch repair, develop lymphomas and intestinal adenomas, although they do not show MSI[35]. The intestinal adenomas appear to be caused by mutation in the *Apc* gene, suggesting that one of the targets of *Msh6* mutation is *Apc*. Homozygous mice in *Msh2* mutation, on the other hand, do not cause any intestinal tumours even after 6 months of age, despite the fact that they show MSI[36]. Likewise, mutation in *Mlh1*, another gene involved in DNA mismatch repair, can cause gastrointestinal adenomas (and carcinomas; see below) in both heterozygotes and homozygotes. When introduced into Apc^{1638N} mice, *Mlh1* mutation increased the polyp multiplicity 40–100-fold, due to substitution and frameshift mutations in the remaining *Apc* allele[37,38].

When homozygous *Msh6* mutation is introduced into Apc^{1638N} mice, intestinal tumour multiplicity increases 6–7-fold with base substitution mutations in the remaining *Apc* allele, although *Msh3* mutation introduced into Apc^{1638N} mice does not affect tumour multiplicity[39]. However, if *Msh3* mutation is added to Apc^{1638N} mice with *Msh6* mutation ($Apc^{+/1638N}$ $Msh3^{-/-}$ $Msh6^{-/-}$), intestinal tumour multiplicity increases because of truncation mutations in the remaining *Apc* allele due to base substitutions and frameshifts[39]. These data are consistent with the roles of *Msh6* and *Msh3* in repairing base substitution and frameshift mutations, respectively.

Stabilizing β-catenin mutant mice

Because APC forms a complex with other proteins that mediates the Wnt signalling pathway, it is reasonable to ask whether mutations in other components of the complex can also cause polyps in the mouse intestines. In fact, stabilizing mutations in the serine/threonine residues of β-catenin have been identified in a subpopulation of colon cancer that do not carry *APC* mutations. To test such a possibility experimentally, conditional stabilizing β-catenin mutations have been introduced that are specifically expressed in the intestines. When expression of stabilized β-catenin is induced from calbindin promoter, mice developed only a few polyps in the small intestine[40]. In contrast, expression of Cre recombinase driven by cytokeratin 19 (K19) or fatty acid binding protein (FABP) gene promoter to introduce floxed stabilizing mutation in the β-catenin gene, caused formation of 700–3000 polyps in the small intestine[41]. These results confirm the role of Wnt signalling activation in polyp formation, and indicate that polyps are initiated essentially in the rapidly multiplying cells in the proliferative zone. The floxed β-catenin mutant mice have been used in several other organ systems, providing evidence for the roles of Wnt signalling in prostate tumorigenesis[42], and embryonic and immune system development[43,44].

MOUSE MODELS FOR COLON CANCER

While all *Apc* mutant mice develop adenomatous polyps, they do not progress into invasive or metastatic adenocarcinomas at a significant frequency. Because of the heavy tumour load in the small intestine, most *Apc* mutant mice die young (4–5 months) due to anaemia and cachexia, and some of them by intestinal intussusception. If additional mutations are introduced into these mice, however, the intestinal polyposis phenotypes are modified, and sometimes markedly malignant adenocarcinomas develop.

Mouse models for HNPCC

As described earlier, single homozygous mutations in the DNA mismatch repair genes rarely cause adenocarcinomas in the mouse. Interestingly, compound mutant mice of some of these genes can cause adenocarcinomas of the intestines. However, their histopathology is much milder than human colorectal cancer, and no metastasis to the liver or lymph node is observed.

Additional mutations in *Apc*^{Min} mice, *Apc*$^{\Delta716}$ mice or *Apc*^{1638N} mice

For example, we have introduced *Smad4* mutation (see above) into the *Apc*$^{\Delta716}$ polyposis mice, and constructed a model for malignant adenocarcinoma[45]. Although human homologues *SMAD4* and *APC* are on separate chromosomes, the mouse genes are both found on mouse Chr 18, about 30 cM (centimorgans) apart. Because polyps are initiated by *Apc* LOH in *Apc*$^{\Delta716}$ intestines, and because this LOH is caused by loss of the entire Chr 18 due to recombination at the ribosomal DNA locus near the centromere, LOH of *Apc* also results in LOH at *Smad4*. Taking advantage of this fact, we have constructed mice that carried *Apc*$^{\Delta716}$ and *Smad4* mutations on the same chromosome in the *cis*-configuration. In the intestinal polyps, both *Apc* and *Smad4* loci are lost, resulting in homozygous mutant cells for both loci. Importantly, the intestinal polyps in these mice progress rapidly into very invasive adenocarcinomas[45]. Interestingly, however, these adenocarcinomas do not metastasize during the short lifespan of these mice. The histopathology is somewhat similar to that of the right side colon cancer in human that is often caused by mutations in the type II receptor for transforming growth factor beta (TGF-β). This model verifies tumour progression by sequential mutations in multiple genes. Moreover, some of these mice also develop adenocarcinomas at the duodenal papilla of Vater, which is one of the complications in human FAP after the colectomy operation.

Colon cancer models with mutations in other genes

Other colon cancer models have been reported that are caused by mutations in various other genes. For example, a knockout mutation in the TGF-β_1 gene (*Tgfb1*) introduced into *Rag2* mutant mice causes adenocarcinomas with strong local invasions[46]. On the other hand, it has been reported that the homozygous mutant in *Smad3,* encoding another cellular signalling molecule in the TGF-β pathway and a partner of SMAD4, develops colon cancer that metastasizes to the draining lymph nodes[47]. However, the penetrance of this phenotype appears to be low, and lymph node metastasis has not been found in all affected mice. Furthermore, the metastatic phenotype has not been observed in any similar knockout mutants of *Smad4* constructed by other groups[48].

With the use of the promoter for the villin gene, whose expression is specific to the intestinal epithelium, transgenic mice have been constructed that express activated mutant of K-*ras* (K-*ras*^{V12G}). Most transgenic mice develop single or multiple lesions, ranging from microadenomas to invasive adenocarcinomas, without mutations in *Apc*[49]. Like in the *cis*-compound *Apc*$^{\Delta716}$*Smad4* mutant mice, none of the adenocarcinomas in this model metastasize to distant loci, although the tumours are highly invasive, locally.

Homozygous mutation in the *Muc2* gene that encodes the most abundant secreted gastrointestinal mucin causes adenomas and adenocarcinomas in the intestines[50]. Although the incidence and multiplicity are low, the adenocarcinoma is locally invasive without distant metastasis.

Mouse models for colon cancer associated with inflammatory bowel disease

Colon cancer associated with inflammatory bowel disease is somewhat different from regular (i.e. non-inflammartory) colon cancer. Malignant cancer develops after a long and sustained inflammation in the intestines. The aetiology of the inflammation is mostly autoimmune reactions, and alterations in various immune cells and mediators have been reported. As models for this type of colon cancer, several mutant mouse strains have been constructed. For example, interleukin 10 (IL-10)-deficient mice produce aberrant cytokines, especially interferon gamma (IFN-γ), and develop invasive adenocarcinoma in the colon in 60% of mice by 6 months of age[51]. Likewise, compound mutant mice for IL-2 and β_2-microglobulin genes also develop ulcerative colitis-like disease, and $\sim 1/3$ of them produces adenocarcinomas in the colon[52]. Interestingly, null mutant mice for one of the G proteins, Gαi2, also develop similar colitis and adenocarcinoma of the colon[53]. On the other hand, introduction of dominant-negative N-cadherin causes inflammatory bowel disease and adenomas, but no carcinomas[54].

MOUSE MODELS FOR GASTROINTESTINAL HAMARTOMA SYNDROMES

Hamartomas are benign tumours composed of indigenous components of the normal tissues, and therefore do not show any dysplastic histopathology. However, some hamartomas are reported to progress into malignant cancer, or hamartoma patients carry a higher risk of developing malignant tumours independent of the hamartomas[55]. Recently several genes have been identified whose mutations are responsible for the gastrointestinal hamartoma syndromes[56]. Induced mutations in some of the genes have turned out to cause hamartomas in the mouse. Below are several models of gastrointestinal hamartoma syndromes.

The *SMAD4* (*DPC4*) gene encodes a cellular signalling molecule that forms a complex with SMAD2/3 proteins, and mediates the TGF-β signalling as a nuclear transcription factor complex. In a subset of human juvenile polyposis, which develops gastrointestinal hamartomas, germline mutations have been found in the *SMAD4* gene[57]. Consistent with this finding, the *Smad4* gene knockout mice develop gastrointestinal hamartomas histologically similar to that in human juvenile polyposis[58]. Interestingly, introduction of the *Smad4* mutations into the $Apc^{\Delta716}$ mice causes rapid progression of the intestinal polyps into malignant adenocarcinomas (see above).

CDX2 is a homeobox-containing transcription factor involved in gastrointestinal development and homeostasis. While homozygous null mice are embryonic lethals, heterozygotes develop one or two hamartomas in the proximal colon[59]. Although another paper claims that the tumour in the mutant is adenocarcinoma, no convincing evidence has been presented in either histopathology or its disease course[60]. So far no human hamartoma syndromes have been described in which the CDX2 gene is mutated. Rather, reduced expression of CDX2 is widely found in gastrointestinal cancers. In gastric cancer, loss of CDX2 expression is strongly associated with poor postoperative survival[61,62]. Thus, it appears that *CDX2* plays a role similar to that of a tumour suppressor (see above).

Peutz–Jeghers' disease is another hamartoma syndrome, characterized by mucocutaneous pigmentation, gastrointestinal hamartomas and predisposition to various cancers in multiple organs. Germline mutations in the *LKB1* (*STK11*) gene appear to be responsible for the disease. Several groups constructed knockout mice for this gene and all found gastrointestinal hamartomas in the heterozygotes, although homozygous embryos are lethal[63,64]. Additionally, cancers of various organs are found in the *Lkb1* heterozygotes including hepatocellular carcinoma[65].

Another important gene in hamartoma syndromes is *PTEN* that encodes a protein/PI(3) phosphatase. Mutations in this gene have been found in Cowden disease and other tumour susceptibility syndromes. Although homozygous mutants are embryonic lethals, heterozygotes develop inflammatory tumours in various organs, including those in the colon[66,67]. Histologically they appear as inflammatory polyps, rather than hamartomatous polyps.

In conclusion, many mouse models have been established that are useful for investigations of the initiation, expansion, and progression of gastrointestinal cancers. They are also valuable tools to evaluate various pharmaceutical and biological agents for prevention and treatment of gastrointestinal cancer. Yet one of the key outstanding issues in this field of research is to establish practical models of cancer metastasis to the liver, lung and lymph nodes. Such models should greatly help us find novel measures to overcome colon cancer in the 21st century.

Acknowledgements

I am grateful to the members of my laboratory who have contributed to the papers I have cited. The research programmes in my laboratory have been supported by grants from MESSC, Japan; OPSR, Japan; University of TokyoBanyu Pharmaceutical Co. Joint Fund; Takeda Foundation, and Mitsubishi Foundation.

References

1. Groden J, Thliveris A, Samowitz W. Identification and characterization of the familial adenomatous polyposis coli gene. Cell. 1991;66:589–600.
2. Kinzler KW, Nilbert MC, Vogelstein B et al. Identification of a gene located at chromosome 5q21 that is mutated in colorectal cancers. Science. 1991;251:1366–70.
3. Polakis P. The oncogenic activation of beta-catenin. Curr Opin Genet Devel. 1999;9:15–21
4. Korinek V, Barker N, Morin PJ et al. Constitutive transcriptional activation by a β catenin-Tcf complex in $APC^{-/-}$ colon carcinoma. Science. 1997;275:1784–7.
5. Oshima H, Oshima M, Kobayashi M, Tsutsumi M, Taketo MM. Morphological and molecular processes of polyp formation in $Apc^{\Delta 716}$ knockout mice. Cancer Res. 1997;57: 1644–9.
6. Moser AR, Pitot HC, Dove WF. A dominant mutation that predisposes to multiple intestinal neoplasia in the mouse. Science. 1990;247:322–4.
7. Su L-K, Kinzler KW, Vogelstein B et al. Multiple intestinal neoplasia caused by a mutation in the murine homolog of the APC gene. Science. 1992;256:668–70.
8. Fodde R, Edelmann W, Yang K et al. A targeted chain-termination mutation in the mouse Apc gene results in multiple tumors. Proc Natl Acad Sci USA. 1994;91:8969–73.
9. Oshima M, Oshima H, Kitagawa K, Kobayashi M, Itakura C, Taketo M. Loss of Apc heterozygosity and abnormal tissue building in nascent intestinal polyps in mice carrying a truncation Apc gene. Proc Natl Acad Sci USA. 1995;92:4482–6.
10. Aoki K, Tamai Y, Horiike S, Oshima M, Taketo MM. Colonic polyposis caused by mTOR-mediated chromosomal instability in $Apc^{+/\Delta 716}$ $Cdx2^{+/-}$ compound mutant mice. Nature Genet. 2003;35:323–30.
11. Yamada Y, Yoshimi N, Hirose Y et al. Frequent β-catenin gene mutations and accumulations of the protein in the putative preneoplastic lesions lacking macroscopic aberrant crypt foci appearance, in rat colon carcinogenesis. Cancer Res. 2000;60:3323–7.
12. Yamada Y, Yoshimi N, Hirose Y et al. Sequential analysis of morphological and biological properties of β-catenin-accumulated crypts, provable premalignant lesions independent of aberrant crypt foci in rat colon carcinogenesis. Cancer Res. 2001;61:1874–8.
13. MacPhee M, Chepenik KP, Liddell RA, Nelson KK, Siracusa LD, Buchberg AM. The secretory phospholipase A2 gene is a candidate for the $Mom1$ locus, a major modifier of Apc^{Min}-induced intestinal neoplasia. Cell. 1995;81:957–66.
14. Cormier RT, Bilger A, Lillich AJ et al. The $Mom1$ AKR intestinal tumor resistance region consists of $Pla2g2a$ and a locus distal to $D4Mit64$. Oncogene. 2000;19:3182–92.
15. Taketo MM. Cyclooxygenase-2 inhibitors in tumorigenesis (Part I). J Natl Cancer Inst. 1998;90:1529–36.
16. Taketo MM. Cyclooxygenase-2 inhibitors in tumorigenesis (Part II). Natl Cancer Inst. 1998;90:1609–20.

17. Oshima M, Dinchuk JE, Kargman SL et al. Suppression of intestinal polyposis in $Apc^{\Delta 716}$ knockout mice by inhibition of cyclooxygenase 2 (COX-2). Cell. 1996;87:803–9.
18. Oshima M, Murai(Hata) N, Kargman S et al. Chemoprevention of intestinal polyposis in the $Apc^{\Delta 716}$ mouse by rofecoxib, a specific cyclooxygenase-2 inhibitor. Cancer Res. 2001; 61:1733–40.
19. Steinbach G, Lynch PM, Phillips RKS et al. The effect of celecoxib, a cyclooxygenase-2 inhibitor, in familial adenomatous polyposis. N Engl J Med. 2000;342:1946–52.
20. Oshima M, Taketo MM. COX selectivity and animal models for colon cancer. Curr Pharmaceut Design. 2002;8:1021–34.
21. Chulada PC, Thompson MB, Mahler JF et al. Genetic disruption of Ptgs-1, as well as of Ptgs-2, reduces intestinal tumorigenesis in Min mice. Cancer Res. 2000;60:4705–8.
22. Takeda H, Sonoshita M, Sugihara K et al. Cooperation of cyclooxygenase 1 and cyclooxygenase 2 in intestinal polyposis. Cancer Res. 2003;63:4872–7.
23. Takaku K, Sonoshita M, Sasaki N et al. Suppression of intestinal polyposis in $Apc^{\Delta 716}$ knockout mice by an additional mutation in the cytosolic phospholipase A_2 gene. J Biol Chem. 2001;275:34013–16.
24. Sonoshita M, Takaku K, Sasaki N et al. Acceleration of intestinal polyposis through prostaglandin receptor EP2 in $Apc^{\Delta 716}$ knockout mice. Nature Med. 2001;7:1048–51.
25. de Leng WW, Westerman AM, de Rooij FW et al. Cyclooxygenase 2 expression and molecular alterations in Peutz-Jeghers hamartomas and carcinomas. Clin Cancer Res. 2003;9:3065–72.
26. Takeda H, Miyoshi H, Tamai Y, Oshima M, Taketo MM. Simultaneous expression of COX-2 and mPGES-1 in mouse gastrointestinal hamartomas. Br J Cancer. 2004;90:701–4.
27. DuBois RN. New agents for cancer prevention. J Natl Cancer Inst. 2002;94:1732–3.
28. Oshima M, Takahashi M, Oshima H et al. Effects of docosahexaenoic acid (DHA) on intestinal polyp development in $Apc^{\Delta 716}$ knockout mice. Carcinogenesis. 1995;16:2605–7.
29. Hioki K, Shivapurkar N, Oshima H, Alabaster O, Oshima M, Taketo MM. Suppression of intestinal polyp development by low-fat and high-fiber diet in $Apc^{\Delta 716}$ knockout mice. Carcinogenesis. 1997;18:1863–5.
30. Yang K, Edelman W, Fan K et al. Dietary modulation of carcinoma development in a mouse model for human familial adenomatous polyposis. Cancer Res. 1998;58:5713–17.
31. Mai V, Colbert LH, Berrigan D et al. Calorie restriction and diet composition modulate spontaneous intestinal tumorigenesis in Apc^{Min} mice through different mechanisms. Cancer Res. 2003;63:1752–5.
32. Modrich P, Lahue R. Mismatch repair in replication fidelity, genetic recombination, and cancer biology. Annu Rev Biochem. 1996;65:101–33.
33. Lynch HT, de la Chapelle A. Genetic susceptibility to non-polyposis colorectal cancer. J Med Genet. 1999;36:801–18.
34. Kolodner RD, Putnam CD, Myung K. Maintenance of genome stability in Saccharomyces cerevisiae. Science. 2002;297:552–7.
35. Edelmann W, Yang K, Umar A et al. Mutation in the mismatch repair gene Msh6 causes cancer susceptibility. Cell. 1997;91:467–77.
36. Reitmair AH, Cai J-C, Bjerknes M et al. MSH2 deficiency contributes to accelerated APC-mediated intestinal tumorigenesis. Cancer Res. 1996;56:2922–6.
37. Edelmann W, Yang K, Kuraguchi M et al. Tumorigenesis in Mlh1 and Mlh1/Apc1638N mutant mice. Cancer Res. 1999;59:1301–7.
38. Kuraguchi M, Edelmann W, Yang K, Lipkin K, Kucherlapati R, Brown AMC. Tumor-associated Apc mutations in $Mlh1^{-/-} Apc^{1638N}$ mice reveal a mutational signature of Mlh1 deficiency. Oncogene. 2000;19:5755–63.
39. Kuraguchi M, Yang K, Wong E et al. The distinct spectra of tumor-associated Apc mutations in mismatch repair-deficient Apc^{1638N} mice define the roles of MSH3 and MSH6 in DNA repair and intestinal tumorigenesis. Cancer Res. 2001;61:7934–42.
40. Romagnolo B, Berrebi D, Saadi-Keddoucci S et al. Intestinal dysplasia and adenoma in transgenic mice after overexpression of an activated β-catenin. Cancer Res. 1999;59:3875–9.
41. Harada N, Tamai Y, Ishikawa T et al. Intestinal polyposis in mice with a dominant stable mutation of the β-catenin gene. EMBO J. 1999;18:5931–42.

42. Gounari F, Signoretti S, Bronson R et al. Stabilization of β-catenin induces lesions reminiscent of prostatic intraepithelial neoplasia, but terminal squamous trans-differentiation of other secretory epithelia. Oncogene. 2002;21:4099–107.

43. Lickert H, Domon C, Huls G et al. Wnt/β-catenin signaling regulates the expression of the homeobox gene *Cdx1* in embryonic intestine. Development. 2000;127:3805 13.

44. Gounari F, Aifantis I, Khazaie K et al. Somatic activation of β-catenin bypasses pre-TCR signaling and TCR selection in thymocyte development. Nat Immunol. 2001;2:863–9.

45. Takaku K, Oshima M, Miyoshi H, Matsui M, Seldin MF, Taketo MM. Intestinal tumorigenesis in compound mutant mice of both *Dpc4* (*Smad4*) and *Apc* genes. Cell. 1998; 92:645–56.

46. Engle SJ, Hoying JB, Boivin GP, Ormsby I, Gartside PS, Doetschman T. Transforming growth factor β1 suppresses nonmetastatic colon cancer at an early stage of tumorigenesis. Cancer Res. 1999;59:3379 86.

47. Zhu Y, Richardson JA, Parada LF, Graf JM. *Smad3* mutant mice develop metastatic colorectal cancer. Cell. 1998;94:703–14.

48. Yang X, Letterio JJ, Lechleider RJ et al. Targeted disruption of SMAD3 results in impaired mucosal immunity and diminished T cell responsiveness to TGF-β. EMBO J. 1999;18: 1280–91.

49. Janssen KP, El Marjou F, Pinto D et al. Targeted expression of oncogenic K-ras in intestinal epithelium causes spontaneous tumorigenesis in mice. Gastroenterology. 2002;123:492–504.

50. Velcich A, Yang W, Heyer J et al. Colorectal cancer in mice genetically deficient in the mucin Muc2. Science. 2002;295:1726–9.

51. Berg DJ, Davidson N, Kühn, R et al. Enterocolitis and colon cancer in interleukin-10-deficient mice are associated with aberrant cytokine production and CD4+ TH1-like responses. J Clin Invest. 1996;98:1010–20.

52. Shah SA, Simplson SJ, Brown LF et al. Development of colonic adenocarcinomas in a mouse model of ulcerative colitis. Inflamm Bowel Dis. 1998;4:196–202.

53. Rudolph U, Finegold MJ, Rich SS et al. Ulcerative colitis and adenocarcinoma of the colon in Gαi2-deficient mice. Nat Genet. 1995;10:143–50.

54. Hermiston ML, Gordon JI. Inflammatory bowel disease and adenomas in mice expressing a dominant negative N-cadherin. Science. 1995;270:1203–7.

55. Haggitt RC, Reid BJ. Hereditary gastrointestinal polyposis syndromes. Am J Surg Pathol. 1986;10:871–87.

56. Eng C, Peacocke M. *PTEN* and inherited hamartoma-cancer syndromes. Nat Genet. 1998; 19:223.

57. Howe JR, Roth S, Ringold JC et al. Mutations in the *SMAD4/DPC4* gene in juvenile polyposis. Science. 1998;280:1086 8.

58. Takaku K, Miyoshi H, Matsunaga A, Oshima M, Sasaki N, Taketo MM. Gastric and duodenal polyps in *Smad4* (*Dpc4*) knockout mice. Cancer Res. 1999;59:6113–17.

59. Tamai Y, Nakajima R, Ishikawa T, Takaku K, Seldin MF, Taketo MM. Colonic hamartoma development by anomalous duplication in *Cdx2* knockout mice. Cancer Res. 1999;59: 2965–70.

60. Chawengsaksophak K, James R, Hammond VE, Kontgen F, Beck F. Homeosis and intestinal tumours in *Cdx2* mutant mice. Nature. 1997;386:84–7.

61. Seno, H, Oshima, M, Taniguchi, M et al. CDX2 expression in the stomach with intestinal metaplasia and intestinal-type cancer: prognostic implications. Int J Oncol. 2002;21:769–74.

62. Mizoshita T, Tsukamoto T, Nakanishi H et al. Expression of Cdx2 and the phenotype of advanced gastric cancers: relationship with prognosis. J Cancer Clin Oncol. 2003;129:727–34.

63. Miyoshi H, Nakau M, Ishikawa T, Seldin MF, Oshima M, Taketo MM. Gastrointestinal hamartomatous polyposis in *Lkb1* heterozygous knockout mice. Cancer Res. 2002;62: 2261–6.

64. Rossi DJ, Ylikorkala A, Korsisaari N et al. Induction of cyclooxygenase-2 in a mouse model of Peutz-Jeghers polyposis. Proc Natl Acad Sci USA. 2002;99:12327–32.

65. Nakau M, Miyoshi H, Seldin MF, Imamura M, Oshima M, Taketo MM. Hepatocellular carcinoma caused by loss of heterozygosity in *Lkb1* gene knockout mice. Cancer Res. 2002; 62:4549–53.

66. di Cristofano A, Pesce B, Cordon-Cardo C, Pandolfi PP. *Pten* is essential for embryonic development and tumor suppression. Nat Genet. 1998;19:348–55.
67. Podsypanina K, Ellenson LH, Nemes A et al. Mutation of *Pten/Mmac1* in mice causes neoplasia in multiple organ systems. Proc Natl Acad Sci USA. 1999;16:1563–8.

2
Surgical strategies in oesophageal cancer

J. R. SIEWERT and B. H. A. VON RAHDEN

PRETREATMENT STAGING AND RISK ANALYSIS

Surgical strategies for treatment of oesophageal cancer are based on exact pretreatment staging and analysis of the individual patient's risk for surgery[1-3].

The most important issue of the preoperative diagnostic work-up is differentiation between oesophageal squamous cell cancer (SCC) and adenocarcinoma (AC), which comprise entirely different entities[4]: *Squamous cell cancers* originate in any localization of the oesophagus (cervical, supra- and infracarinal) and tobacco/alcohol abuse are the main risk factors. *Adenocarcinomas*, by contrast, are predominantly Barrett's carcinomas, arising in the distal oesophagus (within the precancerous Barrett's oesophagus) under the chronically damaging effect of gastro-oesophageal reflux.

Macroscopic evaluation by means of flexible endoscopy is performed and biopsies are retrieved to establish the histopathological diagnosis ('gold standard'). The second important aspect of the diagnostic work-up is exclusion of distant metastases, because only oesophageal cancers prior to systemic generalization of the disease are amenable to surgical resection. In recent years positron emission tomography with 18-fluorodesoxyglucose ([18]FDG-PET) has been established as a very useful and reliable tool for this purpose – in addition to standard cross-sectional imaging with computed tomography (spiral CT scan). With FDG-PET, distant metastases are recognized by visualizing the increased glucose metabolism of tumoral lesions.

After exclusion of distant metastases, further stratification with respect to multimodality treatment[5] is performed according to the depth of tumour invasion (T-category). In the preoperative setting the T-category can be assessed with endoscopic ultrasound: distinction between locally limited (T1/T2) and advanced cancers (T3/T4) comprises the basis for individualized application of preoperative protocols (neoadjuvant treatment)[5].

Analysis of the individual patient's risk is another very important clue to making major oesophageal surgery safe. A specific tool is established[6,7], and has proven well-suited in clinical practice. The score includes basic parameters of cardiac, pulmonary, hepatic and renal function, as well the current status of alcohol intake of the patient and his/her willingness to undergo a major surgical procedure.

THERAPEUTIC STRATEGIES

Different therapeutic concepts are applied to oesophageal squamous cell cancer and Barrett's adenocarcinoma.

In *oesophageal squamous cell cancers*, neoadjuvant treatment plays a major role[5]. These tumours grow in the immediate neighbourhood of the tracheobronchial system, which makes achieving the aim to gain local tumour control by means of surgery alone very difficult. Multimodal treatment is nowadays performed in the majority of cases, aiming at down-sizing the tumour or down-staging the disease[8]. This improves the probability of achieving an R0 situation on subsequent surgical resection. Irradiation (RTx) is used in combination with 5-FU, which serves as a so-called radiosensitizer (RCTx). One associated problem is immunosuppression[9], which increases the patient's risk during subsequent surgical resection. This issue has been addressed with introduction of modern concepts of 'safety surgery'. Surgical procedures are performed in a two-step fashion with resection and delayed reconstruction after a recreation period of the patient[10].

In *Barrett's cancer*, it is easier to achieve local tumour control by means of surgical resection (R0 situation), because the tumours lack the close anatomical relation to the tracheobronchial tree. Therefore chemotherapy (CTx, without irradiation) is chosen in the neoadjuvant setting. The advantage in comparison to RTx is that CTx does not have these negative consequences for surgery.

RESPONSE EVALUATION/PREDICTION

Multimodal treatment strategies for both entities (RCTx for SCC and CTx for Barrett's cancer) require evaluation of the response. This can successfully be performed with FDG-PET. Tumours responding to preoperative antineoplastic treatment show a reduced glucose metabolism, occurring favourably early during the course of treatment. This makes the use of FDG-PET a strategy even for early response prediction[11]. Identification of non-responders is possible as early as 2 weeks after initiation of antineoplastic therapy. This information comprises the basis for a decision to either proceed with immediate surgical resection, or abandon the curative strategy and initiate a palliative approach[5].

SURGICAL STRATEGIES

The two oesophageal cancer entities also require different surgical strategies. For resection of Barrett's cancer, abdomino-thoracic oesophagectomy is performed. Reconstruction of the intestinal passage is performed with mediastinal gastric pull-up and intrathoracic anastomosis (oesophagogastrostomy). Prospectively randomized data support this approach[12], and suggest the superiority of this transthoracic procedure over a transhiaital (transmediastinal) blunt dissection. In experienced centres oesophagectomy can be performed with considerably low operative mortality (<2%) and morbidity. Furthermore the operation is associated with good quality of life.

The approach to oesophageal squamous cell cancers starts with the thoracic part of the procedure. Transthoracic en-bloc oesophagectomy (right-sided intercostal incision and the patient positioned on the left side) is performed. Reconstruction is performed by gastric tube interposition with a cervical anastomosis. Morbidity and mortality are slightly higher (compared to oesophageal adenocarcinoma), but in experienced centres the figure is below 5%. Cervical dysphagia associated with the cervical anastomosis is an occasional problem, and may impair quality of life.

PROGNOSIS

Survival after oesophageal cancer surgery has been significantly improved over recent decades[13,14]. The survival rate is better in Barrett's cancer, with a 5-year survival rate accounting for approximately 45%, compared to oesophageal squamous cell cancer, with a 5-year survival rate around about 30%. A major determinant of a good prognosis is response to neoadjuvant treatment[5,8]. The so-called 'responders' to induction therapy have the best prognosis in both tumour entities. Barrett's cancer patients with response to neoadjuvant treatment have a 5-year survival rate of 55%.

References

1. Siewert JR, von Rahden BHA, Stein HJ. Ösophaguskarzinom 2004. Chir Gastroenterol. 2004;20:15.
2. von Rahden BHA, Stein HJ. Staging and treatment of advanced esophageal cancer. Curr Opin Gastroenterol. 2005;21:472–7.
3. von Rahden BHA, Stein HJ. Therapy of advanced esophageal malignancy. Curr Opin Gastroenterol. 2004;20:391–6.
4. Siewert JR, Stein HJ, Feith M, Bruecher BL, Bartels H, Fink U. Histologic tumor type is an independent prognostic parameter in esophageal cancer: lessons from more than 1,000 consecutive resections at a single center in the Western world. Ann Surg. 2001;234:360–7; discussion 368–9.
5. Siewert JR, Stein HJ, von Rahden BH. Multimodal treatment of gastrointestinal tract tumors: consequences for surgery. World J Surg. 2005;29:940–8.
6. Bartels H, Stein HJ, Siewert JR. Risk analysis in esophageal surgery. Recent results. Cancer Res. 2000;155:89–96.
7. Bartels H, Stein HJ, Siewert JR. Preoperative risk analysis and postoperative mortality of oesophagectomy for resectable oesophageal cancer. Br J Surg. 1998;85:840–4.
8. Brücher BLDM, Stein HJ, Zimmermann F et al. Responders benefit from neoadjuvant radiochemotherapy in esophageal squamous cell carcinoma: results of a prospective phase-II trial. Eur J Surg Oncol. 2004;30:963–71.
9. Heidecke CD, Weighardt H, Feith M et al. Neoadjuvant treatment of esophageal cancer: immunosuppression following combined radiochemotherapy. Surgery. 2002;132:495–501.

10. Stein HJ, Bartels H, Siewert JR. [Esophageal carcinoma: 2-stage operation for preventing mediastinitis in high risk patients] Chirurg. 2001;72:881–6.
11. Wieder HA, Brucher BL, Zimmermann F et al. Time course of tumor metabolic activity during chemoradiotherapy of esophageal squamous cell carcinoma and response to treatment. J Clin Oncol. 2004;22:900–8.
12. Hulscher JB, van Sandick JW, de Boer AG et al. Extended transthoracic resection compared with limited transhiatal resection for adenocarcinoma of the esophagus. N Engl J Med. 2002;347:1662–9.
13. Stein HJ, Siewert JR. Improved prognosis of resected esophageal cancer. World J Surg. 2004;28:520–5.
14. Stein HJ, von Rahden BH, Siewert JR. Survival after oesophagectomy for cancer of the oesophagus. Langenbecks Arch Surg. 2005;390:280–5.

3
Neoadjuvant therapy of oesophageal carcinoma and carcinoma of the gastro-oesophageal junction

S. PETRASCH

INTRODUCTION

Neoadjuvant chemoradiotherapy (CRT) in patients with primarily resectable squamous cell carcinoma of the oesophagus is currently not considered to be standard treatment, and is not recommended for routine use by the German Cancer Society (DKG). Currently, the discussion has tended toward the question of whether surgery is actually indicated following successful CRT.

The research group of M. Stahl in Essen recently published the results of their study on definitive radiochemotherapy versus radiochemotherapy plus surgery in patients with squamous cell carcinoma of the oesophagus[1]. Patients undergoing chemotherapy/radiotherapy (CTx/Rx) plus surgery showed a 2-year PFS of 64% compared with a 2-year PFS of 40.7% in patients undergoing definitive CTx/Rx alone ($p = 0.003$). Overall survival (OS), however, did not differ between therapy arms. A favourable prognostic factor was rapid response to treatment.

In a monocentric phase III study, a research group in Seoul compared CRT plus surgery with surgery alone[2]. A total of 101 patients were included in the study. In the group undergoing CRT plus surgery, patients received cisplatin, 5-FU and hyperfractionated radiation. Clinical response to the neoadjuvant therapy was documented in 86% of patients treated; CR was achieved in 21%. OS stood at 28.2 months in the CRT plus surgery group and at 27.3% in the group treated with surgery alone ($p = 0.69$). Event-free survival (EFS) after 2 years stood at 49% vs 51% ($p = 0.93$). The study was ended early because 31% of patients did not undergo surgery after CRT.

As part of a phase II study, J. Ajani and co-workers[3] administered two preoperative cycles of irinotecan/cisplatin, followed by CRT with 5-FU/paclitaxel and 45 Gy. R0 resection was achieved in 91% of the predominantly T3,N1 patients; pathological CR was observed in 28%.

Conversely, in a retrospective paper and meta-analysis, a group in Palermo found a survival advantage for multimodal treatment[4]. A total of six studies in which patients with primarily operable oesophageal carcinoma were randomized to a neoadjuvant CRT group and a surgery-only group, were evaluated. The addition of CRT resulted in a reduction of 3-year mortality by 0.53 (RR; $p = 0.03$). However, the risk of postoperative mortality in the CRT plus surgery group was significantly higher (RR = 2.10; $p = 0.01$).

Assessment

Neoadjuvant CRT is enjoying increasing application in patients with primarily resectable squamous cell carcinoma of the thoracic oesophagus, including outside of clinical studies. Although the findings of the Korean research group do not justify this approach, the study, because of its high 'drop-out' rate, had a significant bias; the data of the above-cited meta-analysis, however, clearly show an advantage in terms of overall survival for multimodal therapy. In addition to neoadjuvant CRT, there has also been increased use of definitive CRT. Here, a reliable evaluation of response, for example using FDG-PET, is mandatory.

Postoperative therapy

According to the guidelines of the DKG, adjuvant therapy measures are not recommended following curative resection of oesophageal carcinoma. M. Armanios et al. published a multicentre phase II study where all patients underwent R0 resection of adenocarcinoma of the gastro-oesophageal junction[5]. Of the 59 patients included in the study, 46 (84%) received all four cycles of a combination of paclitaxel/cisplatin. Two-year survival stood at 60%. Compared with historic controls, this represents a highly significant survival advantage ($p = 0.0008$).

Neoadjuvant therapy of gastric carcinoma

Final results of the MAGIC study were presented at last year's annual ASCO meeting in Orlando[6]. In the period 1994–2002, patients with operable adenocarcinoma of the stomach, oesophagogastric junction or of the distal oesophagus (TxNxM0) were randomized to either a group receiving three neoadjuvant therapy cycles of ECF (epirubicin, cisplatin, 5-FU) and three addition postoperative cycles ('CTx plus surgery'), or to a group undergoing immediate surgery ('surgery') (Table 1)

The research group of J. Ajani at the M. D. Anderson Cancer Center in Houston, Texas, reported on a phase II study of preoperative CRT in primarily resectable gastric carcinoma[7]. Patients with locally advanced gastric adenocarcinoma ($n = 34$) first underwent two cycles of 5-FU/folic acid/cisplatin followed by radiation and 5-FU continuous infusion. R0 resection was achieved in 70% of patients; without preoperative treatment R0 resection is typically achieved in about 50% of patients in the USA. Pathologically complete remission was documented in 30% of study participants. Mean survival stood at 33.7 months. Because postoperative CRT is standard of care in the USA, the authors recommended comparing this protocol with adjuvant CRT.

Table 1

	CTx plus surgery	*Surgery*	*p*
n	250	253	
OS	24 months	20 months	0.009
Five-year survival	36%	23%	
PFS			0.0001

A D2 resection was performed in two-thirds of patients; postoperative mortality was equal in both study arms.

Remarkable results have been reported by a research group in Pisa using preoperative chemotherapy alone in a similar patient collective[8]. Patients with UICC II/III adenocarcinoma of the stomach received three neo-adjuvant therapy cycles of a combination of epidoxorubicin, etoposide and cisplatin. Following a subsequent D2 gastrectomy, patients received three further cycles. R0D2 resection was achieved in 20 of 24 patients undergoing surgery. Pathologically complete remission was not observed but mean disease-free survival stood at 37 months; the mean OS had not yet been reached at the time of publication after 40 months. The 3-year survival stood at 60%.

A second Italian research group treated patients with locally advanced, inoperable gastric carcinoma with cisplatin/5-FU/epidoxorubicin/folic acid supported by glutathione and filgastrim[9]. Of the total 82 patients, 40 responded to the administered therapy with remission; of these, 37 were referred for curative surgical resection. After a follow-up period of 48 months, 25 of the 37 patients undergoing surgery remained alive (68%), 24 of them (65%) disease-free. The mean survival of the inoperable patients stood at 12 months.

Assessment

The data of the MAGIC study are convincing. ECF can be considered the new standard treatment for patients with operable (UICC II+III) gastric carcinoma. An alternative preferred in Germany may be PFL/cisplatin/5-FU/folic acid.

References

1. Stahl M, Wilke H, Stuschke M et al. Clinical response to induction chemotherapy predicts local control and long-term survival in multimodal treatment of patients with locally advanced esophageal cancer. J Cancer Res Clin Oncol. 2005;131:67–72.
2. Lee JL, Park SI, Kim SB et al. A single institutional phase III trial of preoperative chemotherapy with hyperfractionation radiotherapy plus surgery versus surgery alone for resectable esophageal squamous cell carcinoma. Annals Oncol. 2004;15:947–54.
3. Ajani JA, Walsh G, Komaki R et al. Preoperative induction of CPT-11 and cisplatin chemotherapy followed by chemoradiotherapy in patients with locoregional carcinoma of the esophagus or gastroesophageal junction. Cancer. 2004;100:2347–54.
4. Fiorica F, Di Bona D, Schepis F et al. Preoperative chemoradiotherapy for oesophageal cancer: a systematic review and meta-analysis. Gut. 2004;53:925–30.
5. Armanios M, Xu R, Forasteire AA et al. Adjuvant chemotherapy for resected adenocarcinoma of the esophagus, gastro-esophageal junction, and cardia: phase II trial (E8296) of the Eastern Cooperative Oncology Group. J Clin Oncol. 2004;22:4495–9.
6. Cunningham D, Allum WH, Stenning SP, Weeden S. Perioperative chemotherapy in operable gastric and lower oesophageal cancer: final results of a randomised, controlled trial (the MAGIC trial, ISRCTN 93793971). J Clin Oncol. 2005;23(Suppl 16):A-4001 (abstract).
7. Ajani JA, Mansfield PF, Janjan N et al. Multi-institutional trial of preoperative chemoradiotherapy in patients with potentially resectable gastric carcinoma. J Clin Oncol. 2004;22:2774–80.
8. Barone C, Cassano A, Pozzo C et al. Long-term follow-up of a pilot phase II study with neoadjuvant epidoxorubicin, etoposide and cisplatin in gastric cancer. Oncology. 2004;67:48–53.
9. Cascinu S, Scartozzi M, Labianca R et al. High curative resection rate with weekly cisplatin, 5-fluorouracil, epidoxorubicin, 6S-leucovorin, glutathione, and filgastrim in patients with locally advanced, unresectable gastric cancer: a report from the Italian Group for the Study of Digestive Tract Cancer (GISCAD). Br J Cancer. 2004;90:1521–5.

Section II
Gastric cancer: standard and novel therapies

Chair: E. VAN CUTSEM

4
Helicobacter pylori and risk of gastric cancer and lymphoma

W. FISCHBACH

INTRODUCTION

In 1983 the gastric bacterium *Helicobacter pylori* (*H. pylori*), at that time still named *Campylobacter pylori*, was rediscovered by Warren and Marshall[1]. An unbelievable story of success has followed since then, which recently culminated in the Nobel Prize honour for both Australian scientists. There was a clear focus on the role of *H. pylori* in peptic ulcer disease during the first decade. However, it is nowadays well established that persistent infection with *H. pylori* is also associated with an increased risk for gastric malignancies. Within recent years, new insights into the pathogenetic role of *H. pylori* in gastric carcinoma and mucosa-associated-lymphoid tissue (MALT) lymphoma have become evident. The preventive value of *H. pylori* eradication, as well as its therapeutic potential in gastric malignancies, can also now be estimated much more precisely.

H. PYLORI AND RISK OF GASTRIC CANCER – EPIDEMIOLOGY

In 1994 the WHO classified *H. pylori* as a group 1 carcinogen. This estimation mainly came from large-scale epidemiological studies. According to them, and to available meta-analyses, *H. pylori* infection increases the risk of gastric cancer two- to three-fold[2] (Figure 1). Infection with cagA-positive strains is associated with a further increase of risk by 1.6[3]. This association might even have been underestimated because of a possible clearance of the infection in the course of disease development. Taking this into account a population-based case–control study in Sweden came to the conclusion that two-thirds of non-cardia cancers are attributable to a past infection with *H. pylori*[4]. In a recent study from Germany the hypothesis of an underestimation of cancer risk was further addressed in a case–control study with serological assessment of *H. pylori* infection in which various exclusion criteria were used to minimize potential bias from this. By doing this the odds ratio of non-cardia gastric cancer increased to 18% for any *H. pylori* infection and to 28% for CagA-positive infection[5].

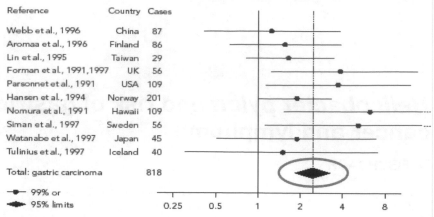

Figure 1 *Helicobacter pylori* and risk of gastric cancer: meta-analysis of prospective case–control studies[2]

H. PYLORI AND RISK OF GASTRIC CANCER – FURTHER EVIDENCE FOR AN ASSOCIATION

There are several other arguments for a pathogenetic role of *H. pylori* in the develop-ment of gastric cancer; they are summarized in Table 1. *H. pylori* infection causes gastric mucosal atrophy and intestinal metaplasia, both known to increase cancer risk. *H. pylori* infection leads to a decrease of gastric ascorbin acid concentration which functions as a radical scavenger. Eradication of the bacterium is followed by a normalization of the ascorbic acid level. *H. pylori* induces hyperproliferation of the gastric mucosa. Hyperproliferation can be regularly observed in the early steps of carcinogenesis. Finally, there is good evidence for a causal relationship between *H. pylori* and gastric cancer from animal studies and experimental data.

Table 1 Evidence for an association of *Helicobacter pylori* and gastric cancer

Epidemiology
Induction of gastritis, atrophy, intestinal metaplasia
Ascorbic acid
Hyperproliferation
O_2 radicals, NO
Hypochlorhydria, hypergastrinaemia
Animal studies
Observational studies
Interventional studies

A prospective study from Japan with 1526 patients diagnosed as having gastric or duodenal ulcer, gastral hyperplasia or functional dyspepsia, and undergoing an endoscopic–bioptic survey over 7.8 (1–10.6) years, revealed cancer development in 2.9% of infected individuals, while all *H. pylori*-negative individuals remained cancer-free[6]. Severe atrophy, a corpus-predominant gastritis and intestinal metaplasia were found to significantly raise the cancer risk. It is of interest that, among the *H. pylori*-positive patients who developed cancer, there was no single case with duodenal ulcer. However, cancer risk was 4.7%, 2.2% and 3.4% for patients with dyspepsia, hyperplasia, and gastric ulcer, respectively.

Two interventional studies have been published so far. In Columbia, which is known for a high prevalence of gastric cancer and of multifocal atrophy and intestinal metaplasia, successful eradication of *H. pylori* was followed by a significant reduction of these surrogate markers[7]. Supplementation of β-carotene and of ascorbic acid also led to a reduction of atrophy and intestinal metaplasia. A combination of eradication therapy and supplementation was not superior to the corresponding monotherapy. A population-based randomized placebo-controlled study recently showed that eradication of *H. pylori* can prevent gastric cancer in a subset of patients[8]. The significant reduction in cancer incidence was found in those subjects not revealing precancerous changes such as atrophy, intestinal metaplasia or dysplasia at the beginning of the 7.5-year follow-up. The missing preventive effect of *H. pylori* eradication in individuals with pre-existing precancerous changes can be explained by the fact that treatment of the infection was too late. Probably atrophy, metaplasia and dysplasia represent a point of no return beyond which *H. pylori* eradication is no longer protective (Figure 2). These theoretical considerations, and the findings of the study, advocate early eradication treatment.

H. PYLORI AND RISK OF GASTRIC CANCER – WHO DEVELOPS CANCER?

The German Health and Nutrition Survey has shown that the prevalence of *H. pylori* infection is significantly higher in individuals with a family history of cancer (69%) than in those without (44%)[9]. This association was not confounded by various parameters. Thus, the familial risk of gastric cancer could be due to an intrafamilial clustering of *H. pylori* infection. In another survey from the Saarland, the same authors demonstrated that *H. pylori* and familial cancer history are independent risk factors[10]. *H. pylori* CagA-positive individuals with a family history of gastric cancer had an 8-fold and a 16-fold increased risk for gastric and non-cardia cancer, respectively. How can this be explained? It seems possible that a genetic disposition (representing the family history) can induce the development of a risk (corpus-predominant) gastritis which increases the cancer risk. There is now some evidence that cytokine genetic polymorphisms may play an important role in the development of gastric cancer[11]. Recent studies linked cytokine gene polymorphisms to *H. pylori*-related gastric cancer development in more detail. Rad et al. showed that

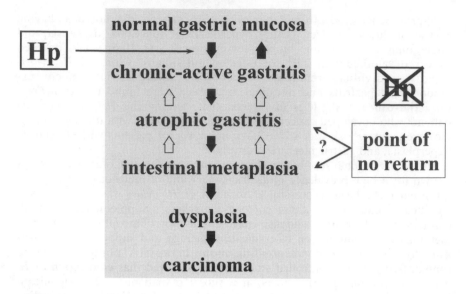

Figure 2   Gastric carcinogenesis, the role of *Helicobacter pylori* (Hp) and consequences of its successful eradication

proinflammatory interleukin 1 (IL-1) polymorphisms are associated with a more severe inflammation and increased prevalence of intestinal metaplasia and atrophic gastritis[12]. ATA haplotype carriers of ILK-10 were colonized by more virulent *H. pylori* strains. In the Chinese population genetic polymorphisms in IL-8, IL-10, and tumour necrosis factor alpha (TNF-α) are obviously involved in the carcinogenetic process[13]. Finally, two recent papers report on IL-1B polymorphisms as predisposing factors for gastric cancer in a Chinese and Korean population[14,15]. Figure 3 illustrates the possible interactions and the players involved in *H. pylori*-related gastric carcinogenesis. Over and beyond this, new aspects of host and exogene factors interactions with potential implications on cancer development recently became evident suggesting that epithelial cancers can originate from bone marrow-derived cells after *H. pylori*-induced gastritis[16].

H. PYLORI AND RISK OF GASTRIC CANCER – WHO SHOULD BE TREATED BY PROPHYLACTIC H. PYLORI ERADICATION?

As discussed above, *H. pylori* infection contributes substantially to the development of gastric cancer. Therefore, infected patients treated by prophylactic eradication of the bacterium could benefit from such an approach in terms of decrease of mortality. However, the effect of prophylactic eradication of *H. pylori* on gastric cancer incidence is at present unknown. Although there is no doubt that elimination of *H. pylori* will reduce

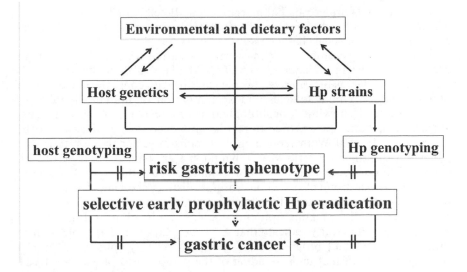

Figure 3 *Helicobacter pylori* and risk of gastric cancer

Table 2 Who should be treated by *Helicobacter pylori* eradication for gastric cancer prophylaxis?

Endoscopic mucosal resection of high-grade dysplasia or gastric cancer or subtotal gastrectomy
Familial clustering of gastric cancer
Risk gastritis (predominant corpus gastritis, atrophy, intestinal metaplasia)
Young patient (<40 years ?)
Patient's wishes

---

the risk for gastric cancer, we also have to keep in mind that broad eradication strategies may harm the population with respect to a possible increase of antibiotic-resistant bacteria, development of other adverse health outcomes and finally costs. We therefore need future risk stratifications to identify those individuals who really benefit from eradication therapy. Currently, in my opinion there is an indication for prophylactic *H. pylori* eradication in patients summarized in Table 2.

H. PYLORI AND GASTRIC LYMPHOMA – PATHOGENETIC CONSIDERATIONS

Based on the outstanding work of Isaacson and Spencer and the establishment of the concept of mucosa-associated lymphoid tissue (MALT), primary gastrointestinal lymphomas are nowadays considered as a distinct entity. This is reflected by the new WHO classification of 2002[17]. The vast majority of gastric lymphoma are extranodal marginal zone B-cell lymphomas of MALT, which can be identified by means of histopathological, immunohistochemical and molecular biological characteristics.

Intensive basic scientific and clinical studies during the past 15 years have dealt with the origin of acquired MALT. In the late 1980s Stolte and others identified *H. pylori* as the cause of chronic gastritis with consequent acquisition of intramucosal lymph follicles and accumulation of immunoglobulin A-producing cells showing morphological characteristics of MALT. This acquired lymphatic tissue proved to regress after successful eradication of the bacterium[18]. In 1991 Wotherspoon et al. demonstrated for the first time that patients with primary gastric MALT lymphoma are regularly infected by *H. pylori*[19]. With a positivity rate of 90% to almost 100% this finding has been confirmed by our group also, demonstrating a distinct association with CagA-positive *H. pylori* strains[20]. In addition to these histomorphological and serological studies, recent epidemiological, molecular biological and experimental data clearly indicate that *H. pylori* plays a decisive role both in the development and progression of gastric MALT lymphoma. Figure 4 summarizes our current understanding of the pathogenesis of gastric MALT lymphoma. The initial antigen-dependent proliferation is of major importance for an antibiotic treatment approach. As long as antigen-driven tumour proliferation is evident, successful elimination of this stimulus may be

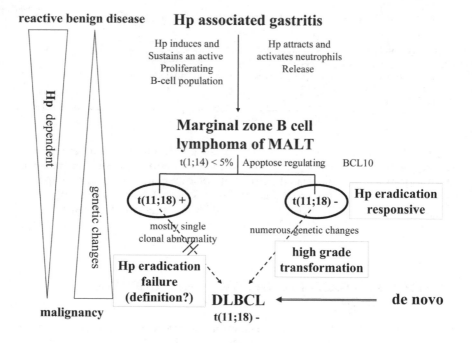

Figure 4   Pathogenesis of gastric lymphoma

followed by regression of the lymphoma. There is a need, however, to identify the parameters for the progression from *H. pylori*-dependent lymphoma to autonomous tumour growth. There is some evidence that translocation t(11;18) is such a prognostic marker marker[21,22].

Obviously some 20–30% of gastric MALT lymphoma cases (see below) do not respond to *H. pylori* eradication. A Japanese group has established parameters that can predict the responsiveness to elimination of the bacterium[23]. They found that all eradication-responsive cases were devoid of API2-MALT1 fusion. Based on a multivariate discriminate analysis it became evident that responsiveness to eradication therapy can be predicted by negative API2-MALT1 fusion, positive *H. pylori* infection, low clinical stage, and superficial gastric wall invasion, the former being the most important factor for the prediction.

H. pylori is associated with a large variability of pathologies such as gastroduodenal ulcer disease, gastric carcinoma, or MALT lymphoma. What are the specific factors that induce the one or the other disease? Genetic differences of *H. pylori* may be responsible for the development of a certain entity. For gastric MALT lymphoma, a possible genetic marker (JHP 950) has recently been identified[24]; its prevalence was 74% in gastric MALT lymphoma compared to 48% in gastritis and duodenal ulcer and 39% in gastric adenocarcinoma. JHP 950 increases the risk for a marginal zone B-cell lymphoma of MALT by a factor of 3. Moreover, JHP 950 forms a gene cluster with ice A1 and sub A 'on' which is associated with gastric MALT lymphoma strains. Obviously, microsatellite instability and defects in DNA mismatch repair mechanisms are also involved in the pathogenesis of gastric MALT lymphoma[25]. On the other hand, the host genetic background to develop gastric MALT lymphoma is still widely unknown. Current studies on genetic susceptibility markers will elucidate this field in the future[26].

H. PYLORI ERADICATION THERAPY IN GASTRIC MALT LYMPHOMA

As outlined above, *H. pylori* plays a decisive role in the development and progression of gastric marginal zone B-cell lymphoma of MALT type. This convincing evidence inevitably involved a therapeutic effort. In 1993 Wotherspoon et al. reported a complete regression of low-grade lymphoma following successful *H. pylori* eradication in five of six cases[27]. Nowadays, eradication of *H. pylori* is considered the well-accepted initial therapy in case of localized (stage I) low-grade gastric MALT lymphoma[28]. However, data on the long-term outcome of patients undergoing exclusive eradication therapy were rare until very recently, and the curative potential of this strategy was still under debate. In a large prospective series of 95 patients with a median follow-up of 49.5 months 59% revealed a continuous complete remission of the lymphoma[29]. This favourable long-term outcome obviously offers a real chance of cure to the majority of patients treated by successful *H. pylori* eradication. Another 18% of patients revealed histologically persisting lymphoma infiltrates despite normalization of the endoscopic findings. Patients with this condition were classified as having minimal residual disease.

stage	MALT	large B-cell-ly
I 1/2	**Hp eradication** if Hp-, progression or relapse: RTx (surgery) **MRD: watch-and-wait**	CTx ± RTx (surgery + CTx) ((Hp eradication))
II 1/2	RTx (surgery)	CTx ± RTx (surgery + CTx)
III / IV	CTx	CTx ± RTx

Figure 5   Therapy of gastric lymphoma

As treatment failures they have up to now been referred to radiation, surgery, or chemotherapy. However, this obviously represents an unnecessary overtreatment. There is good evidence from a large international series that most patients with minimal residual disease have a favourable course of disease, and that a watch-and-wait strategy with regular endoscopic–bioptic controls should become the approach of choice in this condition[30].

It has to be mentioned that *H. pylori* eradication may also lead to complete remission of diffuse large B-cell (high-grade) lymphomas in individual cases[31,32]. It has to emphasized, however, that, contrary to eradication therapy in gastric MALT lymphoma, this treatment strategy represents a highly experimental approach which requires very thorough and short-term controls. In case of no treatment response, early chemotherapy is mandatory in these patients with diffuse large B-cell lymphomas.

Figure 5 summarizes the current treatment strategies in gastric lymphoma of low- and high-grade malignancy.

References

1. Warren JR, Marshall BJ. Unidentified curved bacilli on gastric epithelium in active chronic gastritis. Lancet. 1983;1:1273–5.
2. Danesh J. *Helicobacter pylori* infection and gastric cancer: systematic review of epidemiological studies. Aliment Pharmacol Ther. 1999;94:2373–9.
3. Huang JQ, Zheng GF, Sumanac K. Meta-analysis of the relationship between cagA seropositivity and gastric cancer. Gastroenterology. 2003;125:1636–44.
4. Ekström AM, Held M, Hansson LE et al. *Helicobacter pylori* in gastric cancer established by CagA immunoblot as a marker of past infection. Gastroenterology. 2001;121:7784–91.
5. Brenner H, Arndt V, Stegmaier C. Is *Helicobacter pylori* infection a necessary condition for noncardia gastric cancer? Am J Epidemiol. 2004;159:252–8.
6. Uemura N, Okamoto S, Yamamoto S et al. *Helicobacter pylori* infection and the development of gastric cancer. N Engl J Med. 2001;345:784–9.
7. Correa P, Fontham ETH, Bravo JC et al. Chemoprevention of gastric dysplasia: randomized trial of antioxidant supplements and anti-*Helicobacter pylori* therapy. J Natl Cancer Inst. 2000;92:1881–8.
8. Wong BC, Lam SK, Wong WM. *Helicobacter pylori* eradication to prevent gastric cancer in a high-risk region of China: a randomized controlled trial. J Am Med Assoc. 2004;291:187–94.
9. Brenner H, Bode G, Boeing H. *Helicobacter pylori* infection among offspring of patients with stomach cancer. Gastroenterology. 2000;11:31–5.
10. Brenner H, Arndt V, Stürmer Th et al. Individual and joint contribution of family history and *Helicobacter pylori* infection to the risk of gastric carcinoma. Cancer. 2000;88:274–9.
11. Machado JC, Figueiredo C, Canedo P et al. A proinflammatory genetic profile increases the risk for chronic atrophic gastritis and gastric carcinoma. Gastroenterology. 2003;125:364–71.
12. Rad R, Dossumbekova A, Neu B. Cytokine gene polymorphisms influence mucosal cytokine expression, gastric inflammation, and host-specific colonisation during *Helicobacter pylori* infection. Gut. 2004;53:1082–9.
13. Lu W, Pan K, Zhang L et al. Genetic polymorphisms of interleukin (IL)-1B, IL-1RN, IL-8, IL-10 and tumor necrosis factor alpha and risk of gastric cancer in a Chinese population. Carcinogenesis. 2005;26:631–6.
14. Yang J, Hu Z, Xu Y et al. Interleukin-1B gene promoter variants are associated with increased risk of gastric cancer in a Chinese population. Cancer Lett. 2004;215:191–8.
15. Chang YW, Jang JY, Kim NH et al. Interleukin-1B (IL-1B) polymorphisms and gastric mucosal levels of IL-1beta cytokine in Korean patients with gastric cancer. Int J Cancer. 2005;114:465–71.
16. Houghton JM, Stoicov C, Nomura S et al. Gastric cancer originating from bone marrow-derived cells. Science. 2004;306:1568–71.
17. Jaffe ES, Harris NL, Stein H, Vardiman JW. World Health Organization and Classification of Tumours: Pathology and Genetics: Tumours of Haematopoietic and Lymphoid Tissues. Lyon: IARC Press, 2002.
18. Stolte M. *Helicobacter pylori* gastritis and gastric MALT-lymphoma. Lancet. 1992;339:745.
19. Wotherspoon A, Ortiz-Hidalgo C, Falzon MR, Isaacson PG. *Helicobacter pylori*-associated gastritis and primary B-cell gastric lymphoma. Lancet. 1991;338:1175–6.
20. Eck M, Schmausser W, Haas R et al. MALT-type lymphoma of the stomach is associated with *Helicobacter pylori* strains expressing the CagA protein. Gastroenterology. 1997;112:1482–6.
21. Liu H, Ye H, Ruskone-Fourmestraux A et al. T(11;18) is a marker for all stage gastric MALT lymphomas that will not respond to *H. pylori* eradication. Gastroenterology. 2002;122:1286–94.
22. Fischbach W, Goebeler-Kolve M-E, Starostik P et al. Minimal residual low-grade gastric MALT-type lymphoma after eradication of *Helicobacter pylori*. Lancet. 2002;360:547–8.
23. Inagaki H, Nakamura T, Li C et al. Gastric MALT lymphomas are divided into three groups based on responsiveness to *Helicobacter pylori* eradication and detection of API2-MALT1 fusion. Am J Surg Pathol. 2004;28:1560–7.

24. Lehours P, Dupouy S, Bergey B et al. Identification of a genetic marker of Helicobacter pylori strains involved in gastric extranodal marginal zone B-cell lymphoma of MALT-type. Gut. 2004;53:931–7.
25. Niv E, Bomstein Y, Bernheim J, Lishner M. Microsatellite instability in gastric MALT lymphoma. Mod Pathol. 2004;17:1407–13.
26. Fischbach W, Chan AO, Wong BC. *Helicobacter pylori* and gastric malignancy. Helicobacter. 2005;10(Suppl. 1):34–9.
27. Wotherspoon AC, Doglioni C, Diss TC et al. Regression of primary low-grade B-cell gastric lymphoma of mucosa-associated lymphoid tissue type after eradication of *Helicobacter pylori*. Lancet. 1993;342:575–7.
28. Fischbach W. Primary gastric lymphoma of MALT: considerations of pathogenesis, diagnosis and therapy. Can J Gastroenterol. 2000;14(Suppl. D):44–50D.
29. Fischbach W, Goebeler-Kolve ME, Dragosics B et al. Long-term outcome of patients with gastric marginal zone B-cell lymphoma of mucosa-associated lymphoid tissue (MALT) following exclusive *Helicobacter pylori* eradication therapy: experience from a large prospective series. Gut. 2004;53:34–7.
30. Goebeler ME, Savio A, Wündisch T et al. Patients with minimal residuals of gastric MALT lymphoma after eradication of *H. pylori* do not need any oncological treatment: experiences from a large international series. Gastroenterology. 2005;128:A289–90.
31. Morgner A, Miehlke S, Fischbach W et al. Complete remission of primary high-grade B-cell gastric lymphoma after cure of *Helicobacter pylori* infection. J Clin Oncol. 2001;19:2041–8.
32. Chen LT, Lin JT, Shyu RY et al. Prospective study of *Helicobacter pylori* eradication therapy in stage IE high-grade mucosa-associated lymphoid tissue lymphoma of the stomach. J Clin Oncol. 2001;19:4245–51.

Section III
Colorectal cancer: the controversy of polyp development – beyond APC?

Chair: J. BEHRENS and P. PROPPING

5
State-of-the-Art Lecture:
The Wnt pathway in tumorigenesis

J. BEHRENS

INTRODUCTION

The genetic basis for the development of several cancer types has been well established in recent years. In particular for colorectal cancer the model by Fearon and Vogelstein suggests that sequential mutations in oncogenes and tumour-suppressor genes lead to progression from single crypt lesions to adenomatous polyps to malignant cancer[1]. One of the earliest genetic lesions in colorectal cancer is the mutation of the tumour-suppressor gene *APC*, which appears to initiate the transition of a normal epithelial to a hyperproliferative cell[2]. Importantly, sporadic colorectal tumours show a high (about 80%) frequency of *APC* mutations. Additional mutations such as of the oncogene *K-ras* and the tumour-suppressor gene *p53* provide further growth advantage to the APC mutated cells and lead to progression to carcinomas. Germline mutations of *APC* are the basis of the hereditary colorectal cancer syndrome familial adenomatous polyposis (FAP), an autosomal dominant inherited disease which is characterized by the development of multiple (more than 100) polyps, which at an early age transform into cancer. Although APC was shown to have multiple functions with putative roles in the control of tumorigensis the main tumour-relevant consequence of *APC* mutations appears to be the constitutive activation of the Wnt signalling pathway.

BIOCHEMICAL INTERACTIONS OF THE Wnt PATHWAY

Wnt signalling plays decisive roles in several development processes by regulating differentiation, growth, and apoptosis, and importantly, stem cell behaviour. The Wnt pathway has been elucidated by a combination of developmental, cell biological, and biochemical studies (Figure 1). Wnt factors are secreted proteins that bind to frizzled seven transmembrane-span receptors and to LRP (LDL-receptor-related proteins) co-receptors. In most cases Wnt act in a paracrine fashion, but may also have autocrine functions in tumour cells[3]. The binding of Wnt to frizzleds initiates several biochemical interactions

37

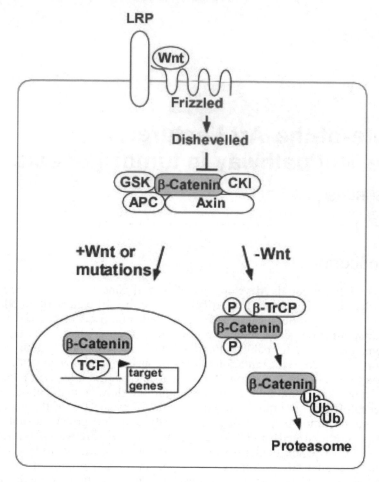

Figure 1 Overview of the Wnt pathway. Binding of Wnt to frizzled receptors activates dishevelled, which blocks the function of a complex assembled over the scaffold proteins axin (or conductin). In the absence of Wnt (–Wnt) the axin/conductin complexes promote phosphorylation of β-catenin by GSK3β (~P). Phosphorylated β-catenin becomes multi-ubiquitinated (Ub) and subsequently degraded in proteasomes. In the presence of Wnt or after mutations of either APC, axin/conductin, or β-catenin, phosphorylation and degradation of β-catenin is blocked, which allows the nuclear transfer of β-catenin and its association with TCF transcription factors (+Wnt or mutations). The TCF/β-catenin complexes bind to DNA and activate Wnt target genes.

within the cell that activate nuclear signalling via β-catenin. The cytoplasmic phosphoprotein dishevelled becomes recruited to the plasma membrane, possibly by interaction with phospholipids and/or with frizzleds[4–6]. This leads to activation of dishevelled, which can then interfere with degradation of β-catenin. Direct binding of axin, a negative regulator of β-catenin stability, to the frizzled co-receptor LRP has also been demonstrated and likewise associated with the reduced degradation of β-catenin. Thus, the intracellular signalling cascade originating from the Wnt/frizzled interaction leads to the stabilization of β-catenin and its accumulation in the cytoplasm. β-Catenin can then enter the nucleus where it forms complexes with HMG box transcription factors of the transcription factors of the lymphoid enhancer factor/T-cell factor (LEF/TCF) family (referred to below as TCF[7–9]). TCF bind to DNA via an HMG domain and to β-catenin with a short stretch of amino acids at their N-terminus. TCF lack transactivation function; however, in β-catenin, the N-terminal, and in particular the C-terminal, regions that flank a central armadillo repeat domain exhibit transcriptional activation function. After binding to specific promoter elements the TCF/β-catenin complexes activate target genes together with co-activators such as SWI/SNF and p300/CBP[10,11]. The nuclear import of β-catenin does not require a nuclear-localization signal and is independent of importins, but depends on binding to legless/Bcl-9 and pygopus co-factors[12–14]. β-Catenin can also interact with the cytoplasmic domain of cadherins, and provides a link to the actin cytoskeleton via its binding to the vinculin-related protein α-catenin[15]. It is not yet clear to what degree the cell adhesion function of β-catenin plays a role in Wnt signalling, but it is well established from many studies that disturbances of cell junctions is a prerequisite for tumour invasion and metastasis.

APC acts as a strong negative regulator of the Wnt pathway by inducing degradation of β-catenin in 26S proteasomes[16]. APC is part of a β-catenin destruction complex which includes the scaffold proteins axin or conductin/axin2, casein kinase I (CKI) and glycogen synthase kinase3β (GSK3β)[17–21]. Within this complex β-catenin is sequentially phosphorylated by CKI and GSK3β at specific serine and threonine residues in its aminoterminus[21,22]. Phosphorylated β-catenin is ubiquitinated by the E3 ubiquitin ligase β-TrCP and subsequently degraded in proteasomes[23,24]. The functional role of APC within the destruction complex is not clear. APC can bind to β-catenin via repeated sequences in its middle part, and thereby appears to efficiently recruit β-catenin to the complex. In addition, APC has three so-called SAMP repeats by which it interacts with axin and conductin. The phosphorylation of β-catenin by GSK3β is far more efficient in the presence of axin than in its absence, and overexpression of axin/conductin promotes the degradation of β-catenin[18,20].

Axin and conductin are 45% identical in their amino acid sequences and have similar biochemical functions, but they differ in their regulation. While axin is ubiquitously expressed during embryonic development and in the adult, conductin seems to be specifically expressed in tissues characterized by active Wnt signalling[25,26]. Moreover, in contrast to axin, conductin is strongly up-regulated in colon, liver, and ovarian tumours[25,27,28]. Biochemical experiments demonstrate that conductin is a direct target of the Wnt pathway that acts in a negative feedback mechanism[25,28] (M. Reichel and J. Behrens, unpublished data). Thus, axin seems to represent the constitutive component of the β-catenin destruction complex, while axin2/conductin is inducible. Whether the up-regulation of axin2/conductin in tumours has a functional role remains to be determined. In the absence of wild-type APC, or when β-catenin is mutated, axin or conductin seem to be incapable of blocking the accumulation of β-catenin, but they might be able to retain β-catenin in the cytoplasm to some extent and thus attenuate the signal[29]. Recently we have obtained evidence that overexpression of conductin can induce chromosomal instability in colorectal tumour cells by modulating the mitotic spindle checkpoint (M. Hadjihannas and J. Behrens, unpublished data).

The precise activation mechanism of dishevelled, as well as its function in the stabilization of β-catenin, is not known, but it appears that dishevelled directly interferes with the β-catenin destruction complex[4]. In addition to dishevelled, axin is also recruited to the plasma membrane by binding to LRP, which blocks function of the β-catenin destruction complex[30,31].

MUTATIONAL ACTIVATION OF Wnt SIGNALLING IN CANCER

Mutations in components of the β-catenin destruction complex have been identified in a variety of tumour types. In general these mutations prevent efficient degradation of β-catenin and thereby lead to its aberrant stabilization and constitutive activation of TCF/β-catenin target genes. The essential finding that led to the addition of the Wnt pathway to the list of cancer-relevant signalling pathways was the discovery of mutations of APC or β-catenin in colorectal cancer, and later in other tumour types. In colorectal cancer mutations of APC are predominant. These mutations lead to frameshifts or stop codons approximately in the middle part of the coding sequence, resulting in the generation of truncated APC proteins. As a result the 20-amino-acid repeats that interact with β-catenin as well as all of the SAMP interaction domains for axin/conductin are missing[16]. Although axin/conductin can bind β-catenin on their own, it is possible that β-catenin is no longer efficiently delivered to the destruction complex when APC is mutated. In addition it has been proposed that APC acts by keeping β-catenin out of the nucleus, possibly via co-transport because APC can shuttle between the cytoplasm and the nucleus. As truncated APC lacks several nuclear export sequences this function might also be obliterated as a consequence of the mutations[32]. In summary, APC mutations lead to accumulation of β-catenin and constitutive transcription of Wnt target genes in the absence of exogenous Wnt factors[33,34]. It is not clear why colorectal cancer (CRC) cells retain the truncated APC versions, i.e. why cancer-generating mutations do not completely abolish APC expression. Interestingly a special form of attenuated FAP, in which patients develop much less polyps than in the classical FAP is characterized by mutations that are more 5′ and consequently generate shorter APC proteins[35]. This indicates that the truncated APC retains some function that is required for robust tumorigenesis.

β-Catenin is mutationally activated in up to 10% of all sporadic colon carcinomas by point mutations or in frame deletions of the serine and threonine residues that are phosphorylated by GSK3β[16]. β-Catenin and *APC* mutations are mutually exclusive, possibly reflecting the fact that both components act in the same pathway. β-Catenin mutations are frequent in tumour types other than CRC, such as liver tumours, while *APC* mutations are more confined to colorectal cancer. Mutations of *conductin/axin2* occur in 25% of the microsatellite-unstable colorectal tumours. Germline mutations of *conductin/axin2* lead to the formation of oligodontia and, importantly, colorectal neoplasias[36]. Mutations of the *axin* and *conductin/axin2* genes have also been identified in various other tumour entities, such as medulloblastomas, endometrioid ovarian carcinomas, hepatomas and hepatocellular carcinomas (see ref. 37 for a review).

Recent evidence suggests additional autocrine mechanisms involving stimulation of the pathway by secreted Wnt proteins[38,39]. CRC cells frequently express Wnt, and the Wnt pathway activity could be suppressed by treatment of the cells with SFRP (secreted frizzled related proteins) which interfere with Wnt receptor binding. Importantly, the genes for SFRP are subject to inactivation by hypermethylation in the CRC cells, indicating an epigenetic mechanism that leads to a boost of the Wnt signal[38]. Autocrine Wnt stimulation has also been observed in other tumour cell types, in particular from breast and ovary. Overexpression of the extracellular inhibitor of Wnt, Dickkopf, leads to down-regulation of β-catenin levels and Wnt target gene expression, as well as reduced saturation densities of these cells[39]. Wnt signalling might also induce epigenetic changes through histone deacetylation. Expression of histone deacetylase 2 (HDAC2) was shown to be suppressed by APC, and inhibition of HDAC2 with low-molecular-weight inhibitors reduced intestinal polyp formation in the APC mutant min mice[40].

APC has been implicated in various other cellular processes such as cell migration, chromosomal stability, cell cycle regulation, and cell adhesion, which could play a role in tumorigenesis. For instance, truncated but not wild-type APC activates the APC-stimulated guanine nucleotide exchange factor (ASEF) which in turn activates the small G-protein rac and thereby stimulates cell migration[41]. APC is also connected to microtubules, and it plays a role in the correct establishment of the mitotic spindle[42,43]. Disturbance of APC function by mutations could lead to chromosomal instability which is a hallmark of the majority of CRC.

DOWNSTREAM EFFECTORS OF Wnt SIGNALLING

It is thought that the main regulatory consequences of Wnt signalling are based on alterations of gene transcription via TCF/LEF. Many Wnt target genes have been identified that reflect the diverse outputs of Wnt signalling in normal embryonic development as well as in cancer[37]. Here we will highlight only some of those targets for which a role in tumorigenesis was shown, or can be assumed from their known function. Of special interest with respect to CRC development are the regulators of cell cycle progression, *c-myc* and *cyclin D1*, whose promoters are directly activated by TCF/β-catenin complexes. Wnt signalling might also regulate cell proliferation by inducing expression of growth factors and their receptors, such as the c-met tyrosine kinase. In addition, Wnt signalling can prevent apoptosis by up-regulating anti-apoptotic proteins such as the caspase inhibitor, survivin. Survivin is mainly expressed at the base of the crypts of normal colon epithelium and up-regulated in colon tumours, reflecting similar roles for Wnt signalling in the normal epithelium and tumours. Moreover, Wnt signalling stimulates angiogenesis via up-regulation of VEGF (vascular endothelial growth factor) and promotes tumour cell invasion by inducing expression of proteases capable of degrading extracellular matrix such as matrilysin/MMP7 and MMP-26, as well as of cell adhesion molecules such as CD44 and NrCAM[37] (see http://www.stanford.edu/rnusse/wntwindow.html, for an updated list of Wnt target genes). Thus, aberrant Wnt signalling similar to other oncogenic signalling pathways is not only important for the initial expansion of the transformed cell compartment, but might also be involved in tumour progression. In line with this it is of interest that the nuclear staining for β-catenin in colorectal carcinomas often shows a heterogeneous pattern with strong nuclear enrichment at the invasion front and mainly cytoplasmic and membrane staining in the central tumour area[44]. This indicates that high levels of nuclear β-catenin in the tumour margins as compared to the tumour centre play a role in the transition to the invasive state of the tumour cells. The molecular basis for this differential distribution of β-catenin is not known, but it can be speculated that signals from the mesenchyme that surround the invasive tumour cells might superactivate the pathway by unknown means[44].

References

1. Fearon ER, Vogelstein B. A genetic model for colorectal tumorigenesis. Cell. 1990;61:759–67.
2. Kinzler KW, Vogelstein B. Lessons from hereditary colorectal cancer. Cell. 1996;87:159–70.
3. Capelluto DG, Kutateladze TG, Habas R, Finkielstein CV, He X, Overduin M. The DIX domain targets dishevelled to actin stress fibres and vesicular membranes. Nature. 2002; 419:726–9.
4. Wharton KA Jr. Runnin' with the Dvl: proteins that associate with Dsh/Dvl and their significance to Wnt signal transduction. Dev Biol. 2003;253:1–17.
5. Wong HC, Bourdelas A, Krauss A et al. Direct binding of the PDZ domain of Disheveled to a conserved internal sequence in the C-terminal region of Frizzled. Mol Cell. 2003;12: 1251–60.
6. Cong F, Schweizer L, Varmus H. Wnt signals across the plasma membrane to activate the beta-catenin pathway by forming oligomers containing its receptors, Frizzled and LRP. Development. 2004;131:5103–15.
7. Behrens J, von Kries JP, Kuhl M et al. Functional interaction of beta-catenin with the transcription factor LEF-1. Nature. 1996;382:638–42.
8. Molenaar M, van de Wetering M, Oosterwegel M et al. XTcf-3 transcription factor mediates beta-catenin-induced axis formation in Xenopus embryos. Cell. 1996;86:391–9.
9. Huber O, Korn R, McLaughlin J, Ohsugi M, Herrmann BG, Kemler R. Nuclear localization of beta-catenin by interaction with transcription factor LEF-1. Mech Dev. 1996;59:3–10.
10. Hecht A, Vleminckx K, Stemmler MP, van Roy F, Kemler R. The p300/CBP acetyltransferases function as transcriptional coactivators of beta-catenin in vertebrates. EMBO J. 2000;19:1839–50.
11. Barker N, Hurlstone A, Musisi H, Miles A, Bienz M, Clevers H. The chromatin remodelling factor Brg-1 interacts with beta-catenin to promote target gene activation. EMBO J. 2001;20:4935–43.
12. Kramps T, Peter O, Brunner E et al. Wnt/wingless signaling requires BCL9/legless-mediated recruitment of pygopus to the nuclear beta-catenin-TCF complex. Cell. 2002; 109:47–60.

13. Thompson B, Townsley F, Rosin-Arbesfeld R, Musisi H, Bienz M. A new nuclear component of the Wnt signalling pathway. Nat Cell Biol. 2002;4:367–73.

14. Townsley FM, Cliffe A, Bienz M. Pygopus and Legless target Armadillo/beta-catenin to the nucleus to enable its transcriptional co-activator function. Nat Cell Biol. 2004;6:626–33.

15. Hulsken J, Birchmeier W, Behrens J. E-cadherin and APC compete for the interaction with beta-catenin and the cytoskeleton. J Cell Biol. 1994;127:2061–9.

16. Polakis P. Wnt signaling and cancer. Genes Dev. 2000;14:1837–51.

17. Zeng L, Fagotto F, Zhang T et al. The mouse Fused locus encodes Axin, an inhibitor of the Wnt signaling pathway that regulates embryonic axis formation Cell. 1997;90:181–92.

18. Behrens J, Jerchow BA, Wurtele M et al. Functional interaction of an axin homolog, conductin, with beta-catenin, APC, and GSK3beta. Science. 1998;280:596–9.

19. Hart MJ, de los Santos R, Albert IN, Rubinfeld B, Polakis P. Downregulation of beta-catenin by human Axin and its association with the APC tumor suppressor, beta-catenin and GSK3 beta. Curr Biol. 1998;8:573–81.

20. Ikeda S, Kishida S, Yamamoto H, Murai H, Koyama S, Kikuchi A. Axin, a negative regulator of the Wnt signaling pathway, forms a complex with GSK-3beta and beta-catenin and promotes GSK-3beta-dependent phosphorylation of beta-catenin. EMBO J. 1998;17:1371–84.

21. Liu C, Li Y, Semenov M et al. Control of beta-catenin phosphorylation/degradation by a dual-kinase mechanism. Cell. 2002;108:837–47.

22. Amit S, Hatzubai A, Birman, Y et al. Axin-mediated CKI phosphorylation of beta-catenin at Ser 45: a molecular switch for the Wnt pathway. Genes Dev. 2002;16:1066–76.

23. Kitagawa M, Hatakeyama S, Shirane M et al. An F-box protein, FWD1, mediates ubiquitin-dependent proteolysis of beta-catenin. EMBO J. 1999;18:2401–10.

24. Winston JT, Strack P, Beer-Romero P, Chu CY, Elledge SJ, Harper JW. The SCFbeta-TRCP-ubiquitin ligase complex associates specifically with phosphorylated destruction motifs in IkappaBalpha and beta-catenin and stimulates IkappaBalpha ubiquitination *in vitro*. Genes Dev. 1999;13:270–83.

25. Jho EH, Zhang T, Domon C, Joo CK, Freund JN, Costantini F. Wnt/beta-catenin/Tcf signaling induces the transcription of Axin2, a negative regulator of the signaling pathway. Mol Cell Biol. 2002;22:1172–83.

26. Aulehla A, Wehrle C, Brand-Saberi B et al. Wnt3a plays a major role in the segmentation clock controlling somitogenesis. Dev Cell. 2003;4:395–406.

27. Leung JY, Kolligs FT, Wu R et al. Activation of AXIN2 expression by beta-catenin-T cell factor. A feedback repressor pathway regulating Wnt signaling. J Biol Chem. 2002;277:21657–65.

28. Lustig B, Jerchow B, Sachs M et al. Negative feedback loop of Wnt signaling through upregulation of conductin/axin2 in colorectal and liver tumors. Mol Cell Biol. 2002;22:1184–93.

29. Cong F, Varmus H. Nuclear-cytoplasmic shuttling of Axin regulates subcellular localization of beta-catenin. Proc Natl Acad Sci USA. 2004;101:2882–7.

30. Mao J, Wang J, Liu B et al. Low-density lipoprotein receptor-related protein-5 binds to Axin and regulates the canonical Wnt signaling pathway. Mol Cell. 2001;7:801–9.

31. Tolwinski NS, Wehrli M, Rives A, Erdeniz N, DiNardo S, Wieschaus E. Wg/Wnt signal can be transmitted through arrow/LRP5,6 and Axin independently of Zw3/Gsk3beta activity. Dev Cell. 2003;4:407–18.

32. Rosin-Arbesfeld R, Cliffe A, Brabletz T, Bienz M. Nuclear export of the APC tumour suppressor controls beta-catenin function in transcription. EMBO J. 2003;22:1101–13.

33. Korinek V, Barker N, Morin PJ et al. Constitutive transcriptional activation by a beta-catenin-Tcf complex in APC$^{-/-}$ colon carcinoma. Science. 1997;275:1784–7.

34. Morin PJ, Sparks AB, Korinek V et al. Activation of beta-catenin-Tcf signaling in colon cancer by mutations in beta-catenin or APC. Science. 1997;275:1787–90.

35. Fearnhead NS, Britton MP, Bodmer WF. The ABC of APC. Hum Mol Genet. 2001;10:721–33.

36. Lammi L, Arte S, Somer M et al. Mutations in AXIN2 cause familial tooth agenesis and predispose to colorectal cancer. Am J Hum Genet. 2004;74:1043–50.

37. Lustig B, Behrens J. The Wnt signaling pathway and its role in tumor development. J Cancer Res Clin Oncol. 2003;129:199–221.

38. Suzuki H, Watkins DN, Jair KW et al. Epigenetic inactivation of SFRP genes allows constitutive WNT signaling in colorectal cancer. Nat Genet. 2004;36:417–22.
39. Bafico A, Liu G, Goldin L, Harris V, Aaronson SA. An autocrine mechanism for constitutive Wnt pathway activation in human cancer cells. Cancer Cell. 2004;6:497–506.
40. Zhu P, Martin E, Mengwasser J, Schlag P, Janssen KP, Gottlicher M. Induction of HDAC2 expression upon loss of APC in colorectal tumorigenesis. Cancer Cell. 2004;5:455–63.
41. Kawasaki Y, Sato R, Akiyama T. Mutated APC and Asef are involved in the migration of colorectal tumour cells. Nat Cell Biol. 2003;5:211–15.
42. Fodde R, Kuipers J, Rosenberg C et al. Mutations in the APC tumour suppressor gene cause chromosomal instability. Nat Cell Biol. 2001;3:433–8.
43. Kaplan KB, Burds AA, Swedlow JR, Bekir SS, Sorger PK, Nathke IS. A role for the adenomatous polyposis coli protein in chromosome segregation. Nat Cell Biol. 2001;3:429–32.
44. Brabletz T, Jung A, Reu S et al. Variable beta-catenin expression in colorectal cancers indicates tumor progression driven by the tumor environment. Proc Natl Acad Sci USA. 2001;98:10356–61.

6
Role of transforming growth factor beta and Wnt signalling pathways in colon cancer

B. W. MILLER and L. ATTISANO

INTRODUCTION

The colonic epithelium undergoes constant renewal. The lower sections of colonic crypts contain stem cells and progenitors that undergo cell division and then migrate towards the top of the crypt. Evidence of Wnt pathway activation in lower-crypt localized cells suggests that Wnts are important factors in the regulation of cell division[1]. In contrast to these highly proliferative cells, those found towards the top of the crypt cease division and differentiate. There is evidence of Transforming Growth Factor beta (TGF-β) activation in differentiated cells of the crypt surface since these cells express TGF-β, TGF-β receptors, Smads and PMEPA1, a direct target of the TGF-β pathway[2–4]. These data suggest a model in which Wnt regulates cell division in the lower region of colon crypts, while TGF-β regulates cell differentiation at the top of the crypt. However, our recent data suggest that TGF-β is also active in proliferating crypt cells suggesting that it may also play a role in cell proliferation. Alterations in the signalling of both pathways have been implicated in colon tumours and we have also observed simultaneous activation of TGF-β and Wnt pathways in adenomas derived from several mouse models of gastrointestinal cancers. Thus, there may be considerable interplay between the two pathways in controlling the differentiation of the colonic epithelium during adult homeostasis and in the development of colon cancers.

THE TGF-β PATHWAY

The TGF-β superfamily is a large family of ligands that are involved in the regulation of various stages of development and disease. The TGF-β family consists of at least 40 ligands, including TGF-β, bone morphogenetic proteins (BMP) and activins, which signal through type I and type II Ser/Thr kinase receptors (Figure 1). Both receptor types bind ligand to form a heteromeric complex within which the type II receptor phosphorylates the type I receptor which, in turn activates intercellular signalling molecules[5].

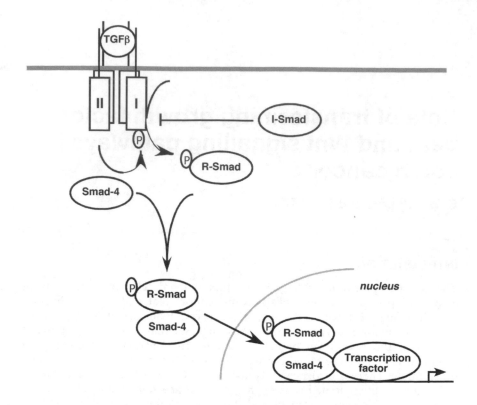

Figure 1 Schematic representation of the TGF-β pathway. See text for details

Smads are essential mediators of intracellular TGF-β signalling. There are three classes of Smads: receptor regulated (R-Smads), common mediator (Co-Smads) and inhibitory (I-Smads). R-Smads consist of Smads 2 and 3 which are responsive to TGF-β and activin, and Smads 1, 5 and 8 which mediate BMP signalling. In mammals there is only one known Co-Smad, Smad4, while Smads 6 and 7 act as I-Smads. The type I TGF-β receptor directly phosphorylates R-Smads which subsequently associate with Co-Smads and migrate to the nucleus[6]. Smads associate with numerous transcription factors and transcriptional modulators, such as CBP/p300 and histone deacetylases, to induce the expression of target genes[7]. The I-Smads inhibit R-Smad activation by competing with them for the receptor[8]. Smads can also regulate TGF-β signalling by recruiting Smurf proteins, members of the E3 ligase family to targets such as the TGF-β receptors and Smad transcription partners[9]. TGF-β can also activate other pathways in addition to the Smads, though the molecular details of their function are less well understood. These include the MAP kinases such as ERK, p38 and JNK, and members of the RhoGTPase family[10–13].

TGF-β SIGNALLING IN COLON CANCER

Mutations in the TGF-β pathway can stimulate cancer cell division, but are also associated with increased metastasis and poor patient prognosis. It has therefore become clear that TGF-β can act as both a tumour suppressor and a tumour promoter.

TGF-β as a tumour suppressor

Mutations that inactivate TGF-β signalling are found in certain colon tumours. Hereditary non-polyposis colorectal cancer (HNPCC) is a hereditary condition characterized by an impaired DNA repair system. In 90% of HNPCC cases there is an inactivating mutation in type II TGF β receptors[14]. Most often a mutation arises in a string of 10 adenines that causes a frameshift or truncation of the protein[15].

Inactivation of the TGF-β pathway can also occur through mutation of Smad proteins. Most commonly, Smad4 has been found to be mutated in colon cancer cell lines and in patients, but Smad2 mutations have also been identified[16]. Smad activity can also be inhibited by other means. For instance, SW480.7 cells do not display an antiproliferative response to TGF-β, even when Smad 4 expression is restored, due to the inhibition of Smad 3 signalling by activated ras[17].

The ability of TGF-β to inhibit cell growth in early tumours has been demonstrated by the addition of exogenous TGF-β, the use of neutralizing antibodies and the employment of antisense techniques[18-20]. TGF-β has also been found to be a pro-apoptotic factor for colon cancer cells[21].

TGF-β as a tumour promoter

While early work focused on the role of TGF-β as a tumour suppressor, it has become clear that TGF-β can also promote tumourigenesis. Overexpression of TGF-β_1 in colon tumours is associated with poor patient prognosis[22]. Further evidence comes from studies on the effect of a dominant negative form of TGF-βRII in CT26 colon cancer cells. CT26 cells are metastatic, but in the presence of the dominant negative receptor they show delayed tumour formation and little sign of invasiveness[23]. This suggests a role for TGF-β in the promotion of metastasis in later tumours. TGF-β can also promote tumours in a Smad-independent manner. In U9 cells, TGF-β down-regulates the cdk inhibitor p21cip1, despite the fact that Smad 4 is not expressed in these cells[23]. Instead, the effect is mediated by ras, suggesting a potential role for regulation of MAP kinase pathways by TGF-β in controlling cancer cell growth. Epithelial to mesenchymal transition (EMT) is a hallmark of the early stages of tumour invasion and TGF-β is noted for its ability to induce EMT. Recently, the polarity protein Par6 was shown to associate with TGF-β receptors and to mediate TGF-β-induced epithelial-to-mesenchymal transition[24].

TGF-β has also been implicated as a pro-angiogenic growth factor. Angiogensis, the growth of new blood vessels, is essential to nourish developing tumours. In colorectal cancer TGF-β expression has been shown to correlate to blood vessel density and the expression of the pro-angiogenic factor vascular endothelial growth factor-A (VEGF-A)[25]. Evidence from non-colonic cells suggests that Smad 3 can cooperate with hypoxia-inducible factor (HIF)-1 in the activation of the VEGF-A promoter[26]. MAP kinase pathways are also implicated as both p38 and AP-1 appear to be important in the induction of VEGF-A expression by TGF-β[27].

THE WNT PATHWAY

A second pathway that contributes to colon cancer is the Wnt pathway (Figure 2). The key effector of Wnt signal transduction is β-catenin. Cytoplasmic β-catenin is an intrinsically unstable protein due to its association with a multi-protein destruction complex. This complex consists of the scaffold proteins axin and APC and the kinases GSK3β and CK1α[28,29]. Axin2, which is related to axin, also functions as a negative regulator of β-catenin[30]. While associated

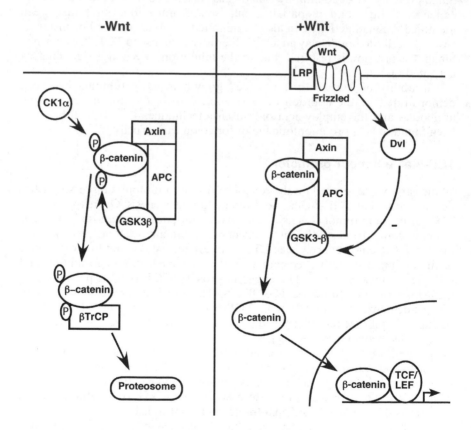

Figure 2 Schematic representation of the Wnt pathway. See text for details

with this complex, β-catenin undergoes an initial priming phosphorylation by CK1α prior to a secondary phosphorylation by GSK3α. Phosphorylated β-catenin is then marked for ubiquitination and degradation[31].

The Wnt are a large family of glycoproteins, 19 of which are known to be expressed in mammalian cells[28]. They bind to a family of receptors known as Frizzleds and their coreceptors, LRP5 or LRP6[32]. Activation of Frizzled receptors results in the activation of a protein known as Dishevelled (Dvl)[33]. There are three Dvl genes, Dvl 1, 2 and 3 which, via an unknown mechanism, inhibit GSK3β-mediated phosphorylation of β-catenin. This results in the accumulation of β-catenin in the cytoplasm and its subsequent translocation to the nucleus. Nuclear β-catenin associates with members of the T cell factor/lymphoid enhancer-binding factor (TCF/LEF) family of DNA-binding transcription factors and thereby regulates expression of target genes.

In addition to the β-catenin-dependent pathway, further Wnt-activated pathways, referred to as non-canonical, have been shown to exist[34,35]. The Wnt/Ca^{2+} pathway is associated with a rise in intercellular Ca^{2+} levels and activation of CaMKII and PKC. The Wnt/JNK pathway is associated with the activation of Rho and JNK. The activation of both of these pathways is dependent on Dvl, but they are poorly characterized at present.

WNT SIGNALLING IN COLON CANCER

Aberrant activation of the Wnt/β-catenin pathway has been implicated as a contributing factor to over 90% of colorectal tumours[36]. However, no alteration has been found in the ligands or receptors of the pathway. Instead, mutations in cytoplasmic components appear to lead to constitutive activation of β-catenin in tumour cells.

Adenomatosis polyposis coli (APC)

The most common pathway component mutated in colon cancer is APC. Over 80% of colorectal tumours feature an abnormal APC protein[36]. The involvement of APC in colon cancer was originally discovered by identification of APC mutations as a prime cause of familial adenomatous polyposis (FAP)[37]. This is an inherited condition, characterized by the formation of a large number of polyps in the colorectal system, and it accounts for approximately 1% of colorectal cancer cases. The disruption of the interaction between APC and axin or β-catenin results in constitutive activation of the Wnt/β-catenin pathway. Mutations that most seriously affect the tumour-suppressive properties of APC usually occur in the central part of the protein that contains the axin and β-catenin-binding domains. Expression of the central portion of the protein alone has been shown to be sufficient to inhibit cell division[38]. A large number of mutations have been demonstrated that result in frameshifts or insertions of stop codons in APC. The most common mutation in FAP patients is a five-base deletion around codon 1309, which is a feature of 10% of cases[36]. Truncations in the 5′ or 3′ portions of APC have less effect as the protein retains its ability to down-regulate β-catenin.

Mutations in these portions of the protein are associated with formation of the less severe attenuated FAP[39,40].

β-Catenin

Of the 20% of colon tumours that are not associated with APC mutations, around half possess mutations in β-catenin[36]. Mutations in β-catenin result in resistance of β-catenin to proteosomal degradation. This occurs through disruption of exon 3 which possesses the GSK3β-phosphorylation sites[41]. Tumours possessing β-catenin mutations tend to be smaller and less likely to be invasive than those with APC mutations[42]. The role of β-catenin may therefore be in the initiation of cancers while APC may also play a role in its later progression.

β-catenin has also been implicated as a regulator of angiogenesis. The activation of β-catenin along with NF-κB downstream of Akt in colorectal cancer cells has been associated with the up-regulation of a number of pro-angiogenic genes[43]. β-catenin may also be involved in the VEGF pathway as VEGF receptors have been shown to interact with β-catenin in endothelial cells[44]. Expression of VEGF-D has also been demonstrated to be down-regulated by Wnt1 signalling through β-catenin via destabilization of VEGF-D mRNA[45].

Axin

Mutations in the β-catenin regulator axin may also contribute to the formation of colorectal tumours. Point mutations in the conserved DIX and APC binding domains of axin have been identified in colon tumour tissue[46]. In addition, mutations in axin2 also appear to predispose individuals to colon cancer[47]. There is also evidence that the subcellular localization of axin is altered in colon cancer cells. In normal colon cells axin is found primarily in the nucleus, although there is a smaller cytoplasmic fraction[48]. In contrast, axin2 is exclusively nuclear. In colonic polyps a redistribution of axin from the nucleus to the cytoplasm is observed, resulting in axin being predominantly cytoplasmic, whereas there is no effect on axin2 which remains in the nucleus[48].

Activation of TCF

Upon translocation to the nucleus, β-catenin activates TCF. The predominant TCF in the intestine is TCF4[48]. While there is no evidence that TCF4 is mutated in colon tumours, it acts as an effector for constitutively active β-catenin. The interaction between β-catenin and TCF4 is considered to be a key therapeutic target. To this end a recent high-throughput study sought to identify natural compounds that could act as inhibitors of the interaction, and two such inhibitors were identified[49]. Targets of β-catenin and TCF4 include cell cycle regulators such as c-myc and cyclin D1 and factors that promote cell migration such as matrix metalloproteinase 7 (MMP7)[50–52]. The induction in c-myc expression in response to β-catenin leads to down-regulation of p21cip1, which results in cdk activation and cell division[1]. β-catenin and TCF4 also induce the expression of an isoform of TCF1 that lacks the β-catenin binding domain and may act to down-regulate β-catenin target genes[53]. Lymphoid enhancer factor 1 (LEF1) is a further member of the TCF/LEF family that binds to β-catenin. While LEF1 is not normally expressed in colon tissue, there is evidence that it is induced during colon cancer[54]. As LEF1 transcription has been found to be induced by β-catenin, it is possible that it is β-catenin activation that drives this change.

TGF-β AND WNT CROSSTALK

Mouse models

There is evidence that Wnt and TGF-β may cooperate in the induction of colon cancer. Several studies have focused on generating heterozygous mice for truncated APC alone or truncated APC in combination with a deficiency in Smad2 or Smad4. When Smad4 and APC are mutated, colon polyps are more likely to form than in mice with only APC mutations[55]. It is unclear whether there is a similar additive effect with Smad2 and APC mutations. One study suggested that mutations in Smad2 and APC do not affect tumour formation, but do lead to an increase in larger and more invasive tumours when compared to mutated APC alone[56]. However, a second study did not detect differences in tumour number or size in the Smad2 and APC compound mice[57]. Unlike Smad2, which is specific for TGF-β, Smad4 is a component of both TGF-β and BMP pathways. Since mutations in BMP pathway components are associated with juvenile polyposis[58], it is intriguing to speculate that the loss of Smad4 disrupts both TGF-β and BMP pathways, and that this might be the basis for the increased tumour formation in the Smad4 and APC knockouts.

Interactions between Wnt and TGF-β pathway components

There are several examples in *Drosophila* and vertebrate systems showing that TGF-β can induce expression of Wnt or Wnt pathway components and vice-versa with Wnt regulating TGF-β family ligands or signalling mediators[59–61]. However, direct interactions between the two pathways have also been observed. For instance, Smad3 can physically interact with axin and axin2. Axin appears to enhance phosphorylation of Smad3 in response to TGF-β treatment and increases TGF-β dependent transcription[62]. The same study also identified Smad2 as an axin-binding partner. This work has been particularly informative, but to understand on a broader scale how the two pathways interact requires high-throughput approaches. Thus, our work is currently focused on using a method known as LUMIER[63] to identify common signalling mediators (Figure 3).

Direct cooperation between the two pathways was first shown to occur at the transcriptional level. We and others examined the regulation of the *Xenopus* developmental gene, Xtwn, and showed the formation of a complex consisting of β-catenin, LEF1 and Smads on the Xtwn promoter. Within this DNA-binding complex, Smads were shown to directly associate with TCF/LEF

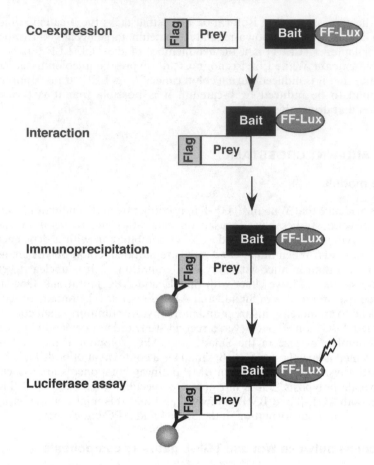

Figure 3 The LUMIER assay. A flag-tagged prey is co-expressed in mammalian cells with a bait fused to Firefly Luciferase. Immunoprecipitation is subsequently carried out using an anti-flag antibody. The presence of the interacting bait is confirmed by luciferase assay

family members[64,65]. The studies went on to demonstrate that maximal induction of Xtwn required activation of both Wnt and TGF-β signalling.

Recent work has shown that cooperation between Wnt and TGF-β in mouse gastric adenocarcinoma cells leads to activation of the gastrin gene when β-catenin and Smads are overexpressed[66]. This suggests that pathway cooperation might also be important in the gastrointestinal tract. Antagonism between the two pathways in the regulation of the c-myc has also been reported, with a TGF-β-dependent reduction of Wnt-induced c-myc expression being dependent on which TCF family member was bound to the promoter[67]. To better understand the nature of the crosstalk between the two pathways, we recently used a microarray-based approach to identify synergistically regulated target genes in epithelial cells. Our results have revealed a complex pattern of independently, antagonistically and cooperatively regulated targets. Of note, expression of a subset of cooperatively regulated genes is increased in tumour samples obtained from mouse models of colorectal and mammary cancer and in FAP patients. Although still preliminary, these data suggest that the two pathways control a specific transcriptional programme that may be involved in promoting tumorigenesis.

CONCLUSION

Aberrant activation of signalling pathways is a common feature of tumours. The role of TGF-β as a tumour suppressor and activator makes it an attractive candidate for intervention at different stages of tumour development. Likewise, inhibitors of the Wnt pathway may make promising therapeutic agents. However, outstanding questions remain about the role of both pathways in cancer. It is unclear how TGF-β acts as an activator and inhibitor of tumours and what mediates a switch during tumour development. There are also a number of aspects of Wnt signalling to be elucidated, including how β-catenin is stabilized in Wnt-stimulated cells and the mechanism by which it activates TCF. The issue of the relationship of the pathways in colon cancer has also to be addressed, as several studies have shown evidence of either cooperation or antagonism. Answering these questions will open up further possibilities of targeting these pathways in colon tumours in the future.

Acknowledgements

We thank the members of the laboratory for discussions. The work in the laboratory is supported by grants to L.A. from the Canadian Institute for Health Research and the National Cancer Institute of Canada. L.A. holds a Canada Research Scholar Chair.

References

1.   van de Wetering M, Sancho E, Verweij C et al. The beta-catenin/TCF-4 complex imposes a crypt progenitor phenotype on colorectal cancer cells. Cell. 2002;111:241–50.
2.   Brunschwig EB, Wilson K, Mack D et al. PMEPA1, a transforming growth factor-beta-induced marker of terminal colonocyte differentiation whose expression is maintained in primary and metastatic colon cancer. Cancer Res. 2003;63:1568–75.
3.   Korchynskyi O, Landstrom M, Stoika R et al. Expression of Smad proteins in human colorectal cancer. Int J Cancer. 1999;82:197–202.
4.   Avery A, Paraskeva C, Hall P, Flanders KC, Sporn M, Moorghen M. TGF-beta expression in the human colon: differential immunostaining along crypt epithelium. Br J Cancer. 1993; 68:137–9.
5.   Attisano L, Wrana JL. Signal transduction by the TGF-beta superfamily. Science. 2002; 296:1646–7.
6.   Maduzia LL, Padgett RW. *Drosophila* MAD, a member of the Smad family, translocates to the nucleus upon stimulation of the dpp pathway. Biochem Biophys Res Commun. 1997; 238:595–8.

7. Derynck R, Zhang YE. Smad-dependent and Smad-independent pathways in TGF-beta family signalling. Nature. 2003;425:577–84.
8. Shi Y, Massague J. Mechanisms of TGF-beta signaling from cell membrane to the nucleus. Cell. 2003;113:685–700.
9. Izzi L, Attisano L. Regulation of the TGF-beta signalling pathway by ubiquitin-mediated degradation. Oncogene. 2004;23:2071–8.
10. Engel ME, McDonnell MA, Law BK, Moses HL. Interdependent SMAD and JNK signaling in transforming growth factor-beta-mediated transcription. J Biol Chem. 1999; 274:37413–20.
11. Edlund S, Bu S, Schuster N et al. Transforming growth factor-beta1 (TGF-beta)-induced apoptosis of prostate cancer cells involves Smad7-dependent activation of p38 by TGF-beta-activated kinase 1 and mitogen-activated protein kinase kinase 3. Mol Biol Cell. 2003; 14:529–44.
12. Lai CF, Cheng SL. Signal transductions induced by bone morphogenetic protein-2 and transforming growth factor-beta in normal human osteoblastic cells. J Biol Chem. 2002; 277:15514–22.
13. Javelaud D, Mauviel A. Crosstalk mechanisms between the mitogen-activated protein kinase pathways and Smad signaling downstream of TGF-beta: implications for carcinogenesis. Oncogene. 2005;24:5742–50.
14. Lu SL, Kawabata M, Imamura T et al. HNPCC associated with germline mutation in the TGF-beta type II receptor gene. Nat Genet. 1998;19:17–18.
15. Paoloni-Giacobino A, Rey-Berthod C, Couturier A, Antonarakis SE, Hutter P. Differential rates of frameshift alterations in four repeat sequences of hereditary nonpolyposis colorectal cancer tumors. Hum Genet. 2002;111:284–9.
16. Akhurst RJ, Derynck R. TGF-beta signaling in cancer – a double-edged sword. Trends Cell Biol. 2001;11:S44–51.
17. Calonge MJ, Massague J. Smad4/DPC4 silencing and hyperactive Ras jointly disrupt transforming growth factor-beta antiproliferative responses in colon cancer cells. J Biol Chem. 1999;274:33637–43.
18. Wu SP, Theodorescu D, Kerbel RS et al. TGF-beta 1 is an autocrine-negative growth regulator of human colon carcinoma FET cells *in vivo* as revealed by transfection of an antisense expression vector. J Cell Biol. 1992;116:187–96.
19. Lieubeau B, Garrigue L, Barbieux I, Meflah K, Gregoire M. The role of transforming growth factor beta 1 in the fibroblastic reaction associated with rat colorectal tumor development. Cancer Res. 1994;54:6526–32.
20. Mulder KM, Humphrey LE, Choi HG, Childress-Fields KE, Brattain MG. Evidence for c-myc in the signaling pathway for TGF-beta in well-differentiated human colon carcinoma cells. J Cell Physiol. 1990;145:501–7.
21. Wang CY, Eshleman JR, Willson JK, Markowitz S. Both transforming growth factor-beta and substrate release are inducers of apoptosis in a human colon adenoma cell line. Cancer Res. 1995;55:5101–5.
22. Shim KS, Kim KH, Han WS, Park EB. Elevated serum levels of transforming growth factor-beta1 in patients with colorectal carcinoma: its association with tumor progression and its significant decrease after curative surgical resection. Cancer. 1999;85:554–61.
23. Oft M, Heider KH, Beug H. TGFbeta signaling is necessary for carcinoma cell invasiveness and metastasis. Curr Biol. 1998;8:1243–52.
24. Ozdamar B, Bose R, Barrios-Rodiles M, Wang HR, Zhang Y, Wrana JL. Regulation of the polarity protein Par6 by TGFbeta receptors controls epithelial cell plasticity. Science. 2005; 307:1603–9.
25. Xiong B, Gong LL, Zhang F, Hu MB, Yuan HY. TGF beta1 expression and angiogenesis in colorectal cancer tissue. World J Gastroenterol. 2002;8:496–8.
26. Sanchez-Elsner T, Botella LM, Velasco B, Corbi A, Attisano L, Bernabeu C. Synergistic cooperation between hypoxia and transforming growth factor-beta pathways on human vascular endothelial growth factor gene expression. J Biol Chem. 2001;276:38527–35.
27. Yamamoto T, Kozawa O, Tanabe K et al. Involvement of p38 MAP kinase in TGF-beta-stimulated VEGF synthesis in aortic smooth muscle cells. J Cell Biochem. 2001;82:591–8.
28. Logan CY, Nusse R. The Wnt signaling pathway in development and disease. Annu Rev Cell Dev Biol. 2004;20:781–810.

29. Moon RT, Bowerman B, Boutros M, Perrimon N. The promise and perils of Wnt signaling through beta-catenin. Science. 2002;296:1644–6.
30. Chia IV, Costantini F. Mouse axin and axin2/conductin proteins are functionally equivalent *in vivo*. Mol Cell Biol. 2005;25:4371–6.
31. Doble BW, Woodgett JR. GSK-3: tricks of the trade for a multi-tasking kinase. J Cell Sci. 2003;116:1175–86.
32. Huang HC, Klein PS. The Frizzled family: receptors for multiple signal transduction pathways. Genome Biol. 2004;5:234.
33. Wharton KA, Jr. Runnin' with the Dvl: proteins that associate with Dsh/Dvl and their significance to Wnt signal transduction. Dev Biol. 2003;253:1–17.
34. Kohn AD, Moon RT. Wnt and calcium signaling: beta-catenin-independent pathways. Cell Calcium. 2005;38:439–46.
35. Veeman MT, Axelrod JD, Moon RT. A second canon. Functions and mechanisms of beta-catenin-independent Wnt signaling. Dev Cell. 2003;5:367–77.
36. Giles RH, van Es JH, Clevers H. Caught up in a Wnt storm: Wnt signaling in cancer. Biochim Biophys Acta. 2003;1653:1–24.
37. Groden J, Thliveris A, Samowitz W et al. Identification and characterization of the familial adenomatous polyposis coli gene. Cell. 1991;66:589–600.
38. Shih IM, Yu J, He TC, Vogelstein B, Kinzler KW. The beta-catenin binding domain of adenomatous polyposis coli is sufficient for tumor suppression. Cancer Res. 2000;60:1671–6.
39. Spirio L, Olschwang S, Groden J et al. Alleles of the APC gene: an attenuated form of familial polyposis. Cell. 1993;75:951–7.
40. Matsumoto T, Iida M, Kobori Y et al. Serrated adenoma in familial adenomatous polyposis: relation to germline APC gene mutation. Gut. 2002;50:402–4.
41. Morin PJ, Sparks AB, Korinek V et al. Activation of beta-catenin-Tcf signaling in colon cancer by mutations in beta-catenin or APC. Science. 1997;275:1787–90.
42. Samowitz WS, Powers MD, Spirio LN, Nollet F, van Roy F, Slattery ML. Beta-catenin mutations are more frequent in small colorectal adenomas than in larger adenomas and invasive carcinomas. Cancer Res. 1999;59:1442–4.
43. Agarwal A, Das K, Lerner N et al. The AKT/I kappa B kinase pathway promotes angiogenic/metastatic gene expression in colorectal cancer by activating nuclear factor-kappa B and beta-catenin. Oncogene. 2005;24:1021–31.
44. Ilan N, Tucker A, Madri JA. Vascular endothelial growth factor expression, beta-catenin tyrosine phosphorylation, and endothelial proliferative behavior: a pathway for transformation? Lab Invest. 2003;83:1105–15.
45. Orlandini M, Semboloni S, Oliviero S. Beta-catenin inversely regulates vascular endothelial growth factor-D mRNA stability. J Biol Chem. 2003;278:44650–6.
46. Jin LH, Shao QJ, Luo W, Ye ZY, Li Q, Lin SC. Detection of point mutations of the Axin1 gene in colorectal cancers. Int J Cancer. 2003;107:696–9.
47. Lammi L, Arte S, Somer M et al. Mutations in AXIN2 cause familial tooth agenesis and predispose to colorectal cancer. Am J Hum Genet. 2004;74:1043–50.
48. Anderson CB, Neufeld KL, White RL. Subcellular distribution of Wnt pathway proteins in normal and neoplastic colon. Proc Natl Acad Sci USA. 2002;99:8683–8.
49. Lepourcelet M, Chen YN, France DS et al. Small-molecule antagonists of the oncogenic Tcf/beta-catenin protein complex. Cancer Cell. 2004;5:91–102.
50. He TC, Sparks AB, Rago C et al. Identification of c-MYC as a target of the APC pathway. Science. 1998;281:1509–12.
51. Tetsu O, McCormick F. Beta-catenin regulates expression of cyclin D1 in colon carcinoma cells. Nature. 1999;398:422–6.
52. Brabletz T, Jung A, Dag S, Hlubek F, Kirchner T. β-Catenin regulates the expression of the matrix metalloproteinase-7 in human colorectal cancer. Am J Pathol. 1999;155:1033–8.
53. Roose J, Huls G, van Beest M et al. Synergy between tumor suppressor APC and the beta-catenin-Tcf4 target Tcf1. Science. 1999;285:1923–6.
54. Hovanes K, Li TW, Munguia JE et al. Beta-catenin-sensitive isoforms of lymphoid enhancer factor-1 are selectively expressed in colon cancer. Nat Genet. 2001;28:53–7.
55. Takaku K, Miyoshi H, Matsunaga A, Oshima M, Sasaki N, Taketo MM. Gastric and duodenal polyps in Smad4 (Dpc4) knockout mice. Cancer Res. 1999;59:6113–17.

56. Hamamoto T, Beppu H, Okada H et al. Compound disruption of smad2 accelerates malignant progression of intestinal tumors in apc knockout mice. Cancer Res. 2002;62: 5955–61.
57. Takaku K, Wrana JL, Robertson EJ, Taketo MM. No effects of Smad2 (madh2) null mutation on malignant progression of intestinal polyps in Apc(delta716) knockout mice. Cancer Res. 2002;62:4558–61.
58. Haramis AP, Begthel H, van den Born M et al. *De novo* crypt formation and juvenile polyposis on BMP inhibition in mouse intestine. Science. 2004;303:1684–6.
59. Yu X, Hoppler S, Eresh S, Bienz M. decapentaplegic, a target gene of the wingless signalling pathway in the *Drosophila* midgut. Development. 1996;122:849–58.
60. Fischer L, Boland G, Tuan RS. Wnt-3A enhances bone morphogenetic protein-2-mediated chondrogenesis of murine C3H10T1/2 mesenchymal cells. J Biol Chem. 2002;277:30870–8.
61. Kim JS, Crooks H, Dracheva T et al. Oncogenic beta-catenin is required for bone morphogenetic protein 4 expression in human cancer cells. Cancer Res. 2002;62:2744–8.
62. Furuhashi M, Yagi K, Yamamoto H et al. Axin facilitates Smad3 activation in the transforming growth factor beta signaling pathway. Mol Cell Biol. 2001;21:5132–41.
63. Barrios-Rodiles M, Brown KR, Ozdamar B et al. High-throughput mapping of a dynamic signaling network in mammalian cells. Science. 2005;307:1621–5.
64. Labbe E, Letamendia A, Attisano L. Association of Smads with lymphoid enhancer binding factor 1/T cell-specific factor mediates cooperative signaling by the transforming growth factor-beta and wnt pathways. Proc Natl Acad Sci USA. 2000;97:8358–63.
65. Nishita M, Hashimoto MK, Ogata S et al. Interaction between Wnt and TGF-beta signalling pathways during formation of Spemann's organizer. Nature. 2000;403:781–5.
66. Lei S, Dubeykovskiy A, Chakladar A, Wojtukiewicz L, Wang TC. The murine gastrin promoter is synergistically activated by transforming growth factor-beta/Smad and Wnt signaling pathways. J Biol Chem. 2004;279:42492–502.
67. Sasaki T, Suzuki H, Yagi K et al. Lymphoid enhancer factor 1 makes cells resistant to transforming growth factor beta-induced repression of c-myc. Cancer Res. 2003;63:801–6.

7
Beyond the adenomatous polyposis coli era: alternative pathways to colorectal cancer

J. R. JASS

INTRODUCTION

One of the practical benefits of an evolutionary model for cancer is to identify the earliest stages that could be either eliminated or targeted by specific interventions. Colorectal neoplasia has been viewed as a developmental continuum that begins with the initiation of an adenoma and culminates with the emergence of a subclone with malignant properties[1]. During its progression to cancer, the precursor lesion evolves in a stepwise manner governed by genetic alterations[2]. Progression of a precancerous adenoma may be marked by growth, increasing dysplasia, and development of a villous architecture[3]. The genetic changes underlying this morphogenesis will be preserved within the end-lesion as a permanent record of the evolutionary history. Since any precursor lesion is usually destroyed by the time a colorectal cancer (CRC) presents clinically, the genetic history as recorded in the cancer DNA provides important evidence of the early evolutionary steps. Associated with this linear model are two central beliefs. The first is that mutation of *APC* explains the initiation of most adenomas. The second is that most, if not all, CRCs arise within a pre-existing adenoma. This chapter will critically examine the role of *APC* as the initiating step in colorectal neoplasia and will then highlight the importance of lesions other than the classical adenomatous polyp in colorectal tumorigeneis. The biochemistry of APC protein and the Wnt signalling pathway will not be discussed.

APC AND THE EARLY EVOLUTION OF CRC

It is generally accepted that the key genetic mutations underlying the initiation, progression and transformation of adenomas implicate *APC*, *KRAS* and *TP53* respectively[2]. Therefore, if all CRCs arose within adenomas, then these genes should be mutated at high frequency in the majority of CRCs. Yet mutations in *APC*, *KRAS* and *TP53* are identified in approximately 60%, 35% and 50% of unselected primary CRCs[4]. Furthermore, only a relatively small subset of CRCs (estimated as 7–25%) has mutation of all three genes[5,6]. *APC, KRAS* and *TP53* are mutated at particularly low frequency in the subset of sporadic CRCs showing high-level DNA microsatellite instability (MSI-H)[7–11]. Genes that are commonly mutated in the latter include *BRAF, TGFbetaRII, IGF2R,* and *BAX*[7,9,12–14]. These facts alone raise serious doubts about the existence of a single dominant pathway to CRC.

It has been widely assumed (based on the model provided by the autosomal dominant condition familial adenomatous polyposis (FAP)) that the precursor lesions for sporadic CRC (at least those CRCs with *APC* mutation) would be initiated through bi-allelic inactivation of *APC*. If this were true, then the frequency of *APC* mutation should be the same in all precancerous lesions, whether early or late. Early, intermediate and advanced precancerous lesions can be grouped as: (1) microadenoma (synonymous with dysplastic aberrant crypt focus (ACF)), (2) tubular adenoma, and (3) villous adenoma. An initial study showed that *KRAS* mutation occurred in most hyperplastic (non-dysplastic) ACF while *APC* mutation characterized dysplastic ACF. However, there were only 20 ACF in this study and only one of these was dysplastic[15]. In two subsequent larger series, *APC* mutation was found in 0/15 (0%)[16] and 4/10 (40%)[17] dysplastic ACF. It is always possible, however, that there was overdiagnosis of dysplasia in these minute lesions. Combining the published data, only 19% of colorectal microadenomas have *APC* mutation. In the case of tubular adenomas with low-grade dysplasia, *APC* mutation has been described in 13/30 (43%) in a Japanese study[18], and only 3/21 (14%) in a Korean study[19]. Only 4/31 (13%) flat tubular adenomas had *APC* mutation in a Japanese study[18]. Higher frequencies of *APC* mutation are found in villous adenoma and/or large adenomas[20,21]. In adenomas harbouring foci of high-grade dysplasia, loss of heterozygosity (LOH) at 5q was found to be restricted to DNA obtained from the high-grade component[22]. Taken together, it is apparent that a subset of early sporadic adenomas may not be initiated by *APC* mutation. Additionally, inactivation of the second *APC* allele may be implicated more in adenomatous progression than initiation.

Even if it is assumed that an *APC* mutation found in a CRC occurred at the step of initiation of the precursor adenoma, then that still leaves 40% of CRCs without an *APC*- initiated step. It has been argued that oncogenic mutation of β-*catenin* could fill the gap left by *APC*[23]. Mutation of β-*catenin* has been linked specifically with CRCs showing DNA MSI-H. However, this association is only with CRCs occurring in hereditary non-polyposis colorectal cancer (HNPCC)/Lynch syndrome (and in only around 20% of these) and not in sporadic CRCs with MSI-H[10,24]. Therefore, β-*catenin* mutation occurs in less than 1% of CRC. DNA methylation would provide an alternative mechanism for *APC* inactivation. In practice this epigenetic change is uncommon and may explain somatic inactivation of the wild-type allele and not necessarily both copies of the gene[25]. Finally, other components of Wnt signalling pathway, such as AXIN2[26] or TCF4[27], include short encoding sequences within their genes that may be mutational targets when there is deficient mismatch repair. However, this cannot occur as the initiating step since the establishment of mismatch repair deficiency must precede the mutation.

CAN *KRAS* MUTATION INITIATE COLORECTAL NEOPLASIA?

If it is correct that *APC* is rarely mutated in the smallest adenomatous lesions that occur sporadically, then their initiation must be explained by an alternative mechanism. There is now strong evidence that precursors of CRC can be initiated by mutations that do not result in direct dysregulation of the Wnt signalling pathway. For example, lesions serving as precursors of sporadic MSI-H CRCs (serrated polyps) can be initiated by *BRAF* mutation[12]. While the related gene *KRAS* has been placed after *APC* in the traditional molecular stepwise model, there are both human[16] and animal-derived[28] data indicating that activation of the MAP-kinase signalling pathway can, like Wnt pathway activation, initiate neoplastic (adenomatous) change in the colorectum. Indeed, activated *KRAS* has been shown to directly influence Wnt signalling in colon cancer[29]. *KRAS* mutation has been found in as many as 63% of sporadic microadenomas (dysplastic ACF) (none of which had mutation of *APC*)[16]. This figure is higher than the frequency of *KRAS* mutation detected in small tubular adenoma (10.6%)[30]. Only in adenomas that are large (>2 cm), show severe dysplasia, or include villous components does the frequency of *KRAS* mutation (29%, 32%, and 28% respectively) approach that of CRC[30]. *KRAS* appears to be highly pleiotropic given that mutation is linked not only with adenomatous lesions but also with non-dysplastic aberrant crypt foci[15], hyperplastic polyps[31], and serrated adenomas[32]. This pleiotropism is explained by the fact that activated Ras influences multiple signalling pathways that may have opposing effects (e.g. pro-apoptotic RASSF1 and anti-apoptotic Akt/PKB)[33]. Therefore, the morphogenetic consequences of *KRAS* mutation will be influenced by co-existing genetic alterations that may promote activation of some Ras effectors while inactivating others.

If it is correct that the earliest sporadic neoplasms (microadenomas or dysplastic ACF) have frequent *KRAS* mutation and infrequent *APC* mutation then one must infer (given the higher frequency of APC mutation in CRC) that the subset of adenomas that is initiated by *APC* mutation is more likely to progress to cancer than the subset that is initiated by alternative mechanisms. However, it is also possible that some adenomas do not arise *de novo* but instead develop within hyperplastic lesions ranging from minute ACF[34] to hyperplastic polyps[35], giving mixed ACF and mixed polyps, respectively. *APC* mutation could be implicated in such a hyperplasia–dysplasia transition. Finally, it would appear that a significant proportion of sporadic tubular adenomas is not initiated by mutation of either *APC* or *KRAS* (Table 1)[4,15–17,19,30]. Mutation of β-*catenin* may make up for some of this shortfall[36].

CONCEPT OF A 'THIRD' PATHWAY TO CRC

Sporadic CRC has been classified into two main groups with different types of genetic instability, those with chromosomal instability (CIN) evidenced by LOH and DNA aneuploidy, and those with DNA MSI in which there is infrequent LOH and DNA is diploid. CRCs with CIN have been linked with mutation of *APC*, *KRAS* and *TP53*[37], while those with MSI have been linked

Table 1 Paradoxical mutation frequencies for *APC* and *KRAS* in early, intermediate and late sporadic colorectal neoplasia (see text for source references)

Mutation	MicroAD	TAD	CRC
APC	19%	33%	60%
KRAS	63%	11%	35%

MicroAD = microadenoma or dysplastic aberrant crypt focus, TAD = tubular adenoma.

with mutation of *BRAF* and methylation of the DNA mismatch repair gene *MLH1*[12,38]. There is evidence for a third subset of CRC that lacks both DNA aneuploidy and MSI-H[39–41]. This subset is as yet poorly characterized and is likely to be heterogeneous. Nevertheless, certain features have been highlighted across this third group including: (1) location in proximal colon, (2) predilection for females, (3) a family history of CRC, (4) tumour aggressiveness, (5) a high frequency of mucinous and/or poor differentiation, (6) mutation of either *BRAF* or *KRAS*, (7) mutation of *TP53*, (8) DNA methylation, and (9) low-level MSI (MSI-L)[12,42–50]. Like the MSI-H subset, this group of CRCs has been linked with serrated polyps as precursor lesions rather than traditional adenomas[44,47]. It is therefore likely that at least some of these 'third' pathway CRCs are not initiated by mutation of *APC* but by mutation of either *BRAF* or *KRAS* in conjunction with DNA methylation. The 'third' pathway may also be regarded as a 'fusion' pathway with features of both MSI and CIN pathways. This is discussed in more detail below.

ADENOMATOUS POLYPS: HAS THEIR IMPORTANCE BEEN OVERSTATED?

The modern classification of colorectal adenoma encourages the view that adenomas are homogeneous lesions that differ mainly on the basis of the evolutionary stage at which they are diagnosed. An early adenoma will be small, mildly dysplastic and have a tubular architecture while a late adenoma is large, severely dysplastic and has a villous architecture. Prior to the international adoption of the unifying term 'adenoma' (classified on the basis of the architectural patterns as tubular, tubulovillous and villous)[51], colorectal adenomas were not in fact regarded as a homogeneous group of lesions. The adenomatous polyp (now tubular adenoma) was conceived as being fundamentally different from the villous papilloma (now villous adenoma)[52]. The latter is not only much rarer and more likely to become malignant than tubular adenoma, but probably evolves through an independent pathway. By lumping all types of adenoma together it is likely that important information has been lost.

Tubular adenomas

Tubular adenomas greatly outnumber other types of colorectal adenoma. It can be deduced from a variety of data that an individual adenoma has a low probability of transforming into a CRC. In FAP many thousands of adenomas develop at puberty while the average age at which one of these gives rise to a symptomatic CRC is around 40 years[55]. Autopsy data extrapolated to a fixed Norwegian population gave an estimate of 26 419 adenoma-bearing individuals aged over 35 years. During a 10-year period 656 CRCs developed within this population[54]. Assuming that every CRC arose within an adenoma-bearing subject, it required 40 adenoma-bearing subjects to produce one CRC over a 10-year period. Some of these subjects will have had more than one adenoma, further decreasing the risk of malignant conversion for a single adenoma. Nevertheless, it would seem that an individual sporadic adenoma is more likely to become malignant than an individual adenoma in the condition FAP. This raises the possibility that there are biological or molecular differences between FAP and sporadic adenomas (see above). The Norwegian study also demonstrated a much higher risk of conversion in the case of villous adenomas[54]. Based on the differing age incidence of adenoma versus CRC, it has been estimated that the adenomatous phase of the adenoma–carcinoma sequence lasts for at least 5 years[1]. This would provide a window of opportunity for eradicating adenomas. Most sporadic adenomas do not progress to CRC at all, while there are instances in which the evolution of CRC may occur very rapidly (see below).

Multiple adenomas

One of the traditional arguments in support of the adenoma–carcinoma sequence is that the risk of CRC is increased in subjects with multiple adenomas[1]. FAP would be an extreme example of this rule. However, there are data to suggest that the increased risk of CRC is not explained merely by sheer numbers of adenomas. The dramatic difference in rates of malignant conversion in FAP and HNPCC/Lynch syndrome (see below) indicates that some adenomas are much more likely to progress to CRC than others and that this difference in behaviour is explained by the presence of genetic instability. The multiple adenoma syndrome caused by bi-allelic germline mutation of *MYH* is one example of how a genetic predisposition factor could explain both adenoma multiplicity and accelerated adenoma progression[55]. This is because *MYH* is a DNA repair gene and, when inactivated, there is increased likelihood of genetic instability leading to G to T transition mutations in *APC* and *KRAS*[56]. It is conceivable that the link between adenoma multiplicity and risk of CRC is more closely related to the genetic mechanism underlying the evolution of adenomas than multiplicity *per se*. This suggestion is supported by a longitudinal observational study that demonstrated that adenomas were more likely to grow in subjects with a family history of colorectal neoplasia[57]. It is therefore likely that known and unknown genetic (hereditary) factors will serve to explain why only a small proportion of benign epithelial polyps becomes malignant.

Adenomas in HNPCC/Lynch syndrome

Just as in the case of sporadic CRC, it is possible to observe adenomatous remnants in CRCs developing in subjects with HNPCC/Lynch syndrome[58]. In this study contiguous adenoma was present in 89% of early HNPCC cancers (confined to the submucosa). Adenomas in HNPCC cannot be distinguished from sporadic adenomas in terms of their morphology. However, they are more likely to be diagnosed at an advanced stage in terms of size, dysplasia or villous architecture, are more common in young subjects, and are more likely to be proximal[59–61]. There are reports of interval cancers occurring in subjects with HNPCC/Lynch syndrome who are under regular colonoscopic surveillance[62]. From this observation, together with the fact that adenomas in HNPCC/Lynch syndrome are not especially common and tend to have advanced features, it has been inferred that adenomas in this condition are 'aggressive'[63]. The term 'aggressive' has two meanings. First, each adenoma has a high probability of evolving into CRC. Second, the evolution of the adenomatous phase is accelerated, perhaps being measured in terms of 1 or 2 years, rather than 5 years or more. Cancers that arise from 'aggressive' adenomas in HNPCC are not in themselves aggressive. The reason for the difference in behaviour between sporadic and HNPCC adenomas has been linked to the presence of genetic instability, specifically deficiency of DNA mismatch repair[63]. This would allow pathogenic somatic mutations to occur in rapid succession.

The mechanism underlying the initiation of adenoma in HNPCC/Lynch syndrome remains unclear. As compared with sporadic CRC, *APC* mutation occurs with reduced frequency in CRC in HNPCC[64–66]. The frequency of LOH at 5q is much reduced in HNPCC[65], but it is possible that the second *APC* allele is more likely to be inactivated by mutation than by loss in this condition. It has been suggested that β-*catenin* mutation could substitute for *APC* mutation in HNPCC[67,68], but the timing of β-*catenin* mutation remains controversial. Some have found a high frequency of β-*catenin* mutation in HNPCC adenomas that were MSI-H[69]. Others found a very low frequency of β-*catenin* mutation in HNPCC adenomas regardless of MSI status, but showed a relatively high frequency of mutation in carcinoma[24]. This would suggest that β-*catenin* mutation is more implicated in progression than initiation of neoplasia in HNPCC. One would expect to find more frameshift mutations in a background of MSI-H, assuming that a state of mismatch repair deficiency is established prior to mutation of *APC* or β-*catenin*. β-*Catenin* mutations are mainly missense mutations rather than frameshift mutations[24], and therefore the reason for their selection in HNPCC is obscure. Some authors have suggested that there is a different spectrum of *APC* mutations in HNPCC, with more frameshift mutations than would be expected[70,71]. Others have found no difference in the *APC* mutational spectrum in either cancers[72] or adenomas[69] in HNPCC. My personal view on this topic is that adenomas in HNPCC occur when MMR deficiency and mutation of *APC*, or β-*catenin*, or an alternative gene are closely temporally related within a single cell. The effect of the genetic change would be to cause inhibition of apoptosis. In the absence of this close temporal relation, MMR deficiency will usually result in apoptosis. A close temporal relation will be a rare event, but this would explain why both adenomas and carcinomas occur relatively infrequently in HNPCC (as compared with adenomas in FAP).

Villous adenoma

In terms of architectural organization and cellular differentiation, classical villous adenomas are easily distinguished from tubular adenomas. In villous adenomas the surface epithelium is greatly expanded and folded into broad leaves in a complex gyriform pattern. The villiform appearance seen in two-dimensional sections is in fact an artifact that results from the sectioning of a leaf like fold of surface epithelium. Unlike tubular adenomas that show loss of production of secretory mucin with increasing dysplasia, many villous adenomas retain a basal to superficial gradient of differentiation in which abundant secretion of mucin occurs in the more superficial cells. Malignant transformation of a villous adenoma often results in a mucinous adenocarcinoma by virtue of this retained capacity for mucin synthesis[73]. These observations suggest that tubular adenoma and villous adenoma do not represent a histogenetic continuum but are distinct and separate lesions.

One of the most powerful proofs of the adenoma–carcinoma concept is the demonstration of residual adenoma contiguous with carcinoma. This was observed in 57% of early CRCs in which invasion was limited to the submucosa[1]. However, in this study, one-third of adenomas contiguous with CRC were villous adenomas. Therefore, to prevent up to one-third of CRCs, one would need a strategy that was capable of targeting the villous adenoma. Villous adenomas are distinguished by a high frequency of mutation of both *APC*[20] and *KRAS*[30]. Despite its importance as a precancerous lesion, the rarity of villous adenoma means that relatively little else is known of its molecular genetic features or early evolution.

Impact of polypectomy on incidence of CRC

Another important proof of the adenoma–carcinoma sequence is the reduction in incidence of CRC that may be achieved by polypectomy. While there is wide acceptance that polypectomy does reduce the incidence of CRC, there is evidence that regular colonoscopic surveillance and adenoma removal does not offer full protection from the development of CRC[74]. The underlying issues will not be presented in detail here except to say that they introduce the possibility of alternative and/or rapidly evolving pathways to CRC. Lesions that have been implicated in alternative pathways include serrated adenomas, large hyperplastic polyps and flat adenomas.

Serrated adenoma

Prior to their recognition in the 1990s, serrated adenomas were probably classified as atypical hyperplastic polyps, villous adenomas, or mixed polyps[75]. In 1970 a paper describing the origin of villous adenoma within hyperplastic polyp was ignored because it challenged the prevailing view that hyperplastic polyps were always innocent[76]. In retrospect, at least some of the well-illustrated villous adenomas in that article would now be diagnosed as serrated adenomas. Some mixed polyps are a blend of villous adenoma and serrated adenoma. The epithelium of serrated adenomas has the serrated architecture that characterizes hyperplastic polyp. However, the architecture of serrated adenoma is more complex than that of hyperplastic polyp, with increased branching of crypts, intra-epithelial microacini and, often, a villous pattern. Additionally, the epithelium of serrated adenoma is overtly dysplastic (adenomatous), markedly eosinophilic and lacks obvious intracellular mucin[75]. Nevertheless, immunostaining reveals conspicuous up-regulation of secretory mucin core proteins MUC2 (intestinal) and MUC5AC (gastric)[77]. Therefore, serrated adenoma and villous adenoma share the property of enhanced production of secretory mucin, though this is generally expressed as non-glycosylated mucin core protein in the case of serrated adenoma.

An important feature of serrated adenoma is the high frequency of intramucosal carcinoma affecting up to 11% of cases[75]. While rare, these lesions may be important precursors of CRC and there is evidence that they grow more rapidly than conventional adenomas[78]. Following the recognition of serrated adenoma, it became clear that residual adenoma contiguous with CRC was often serrated adenoma. Interestingly, CRCs with residual serrated adenoma are more likely to show DNA MSI, linking some serrated adenomas with this particular pathway of colorectal tumorigenesis[79]. This link is supported by the shared list of molecular and biochemical features occurring in subsets of serrated adenoma and CRC with the MSI phenotype. In addition to MSI itself, the features that serrated adenoma and CRC with MSI have in common include expression of MUC2 and MUC5AC, mutation of *BRAF* and DNA methylation[12,80,81]. Serrated adenomas that lack *BRAF* mutation may have mutation of *KRAS*, but *APC* mutation is uncommon[32,82].

Atypical hyperplastic polyps and sessile serrated adenoma

There is increasing evidence linking large, right-sided hyperplastic polyps with CRCs showing the MSI phenotype and DNA methylation[81,83–85]. These hyperplastic polyps differ in subtle ways from traditional hyperplastic polyps in terms of their morphology as well as size and location. The differences include architectural changes (exaggerated serration, crypt dilation, horizontal crypts), aberrant cellular proliferation, absence of endocrine cells, hypermucinous epithelium, and lack of thickening of the subepithelial basement membrane[81,83–87]. Hyperplastic polyps with these features are well represented in the precancerous condition hyperplastic polyposis[88]. They also have molecular alterations found in traditional serrated adenomas including *BRAF* mutation and DNA methylation[12,89,90]. For all these reasons some have advocated that the term 'sessile serrated adenoma' be employed for diagnostic purposes[86,87,91]. Since these lesions lack overt dysplasia, and have features intermediate between hyperplastic polyp and serrated adenoma[92], the alternative terms 'sessile serrated polyp'[93,94] and 'serrated polyp with atypical proliferation'[89,95] have been proposed.

Flat adenoma and *de-novo* carcinoma

The absence of residual adenoma in contiguity with most CRCs could be the result of the destruction of the precursor lesion. As noted above, one is more likely to detect adenomatous remnants in early CRC. Nevertheless, there are numerous case reports describing early CRCs without evidence of a precursor lesion[96–99]. These *de-novo* cancers are usually flat or depressed rather than polypoid and may be less than 10 mm in diameter. It is possible that *de-novo* CRCs could have arisen within tiny, flat adenomas. The use of dye-spraying coupled with magnifying video-endoscopy has helped to increase the yield of such lesions[100–105]. Some examples of *de novo* CRC described in the Japanese literature would in fact be regarded as flat tubular adenomas with high-grade dysplasia in the West (when there is no invasion across the muscularis mucosae). Regardless of how these flat lesions are interpreted, they provide an alternative to the traditional polyp–cancer sequence. This is supported by their differing molecular characteristics, including the finding of a low frequency of both APC[18] and $KRAS$[106] mutation in flat adenomas. Gene expression profiling by cDNA array analysis has also highlighted multiple differences between flat and polypoid adenomas[107]. Some serrated adenomas are flat, and it is possible that the molecular background of flat adenomas and serrated adenomas is similar.

SERRATED PATHWAY AND 'FUSION' PATHWAYS TO CRC

Serrated polyps encompass all types of epithelial polyp of the colorectum in which there is glandular serration. They include hyperplastic polyps, serrated adenomas, the recently identified variant hyperplastic polyp described as 'sessile serrated adenoma' (see above), and mixed polyps[108]. Among the serrated polyps are some (notably the hyperplastic polyps) that have traditionally been classed as non-neoplastic and lacking malignant potential. The fact that most hyperplastic polyps have mutations in genes that are linked to CRC and also show methylation of multiple genes linked with colorectal tumorigenesis means that the traditional view of these lesions needs to be revised. However, this does not mean that hyperplastic polyps frequently become malignant. It is likely that a significantly increased risk of malignancy applies only when certain features are present. These features include large polyp size, proximal location, multiplicity and the morphological findings associated with the variant lesion sessile serrated adenoma[108].

The serrated phenotype probably occurs through inhibition of apoptosis but is also characterized by an altered repertoire of cellular differentiation that could be described as trans-differentiation or metaplasia[108]. When the serrated pathway culminates in CRC with MSI-H status, the evolutionary steps do not implicate the traditional CRC genes (see above). The precursor lesions of the MSI-H pathway may therefore be placed at an extreme end of the precancerous polyp spectrum. At the other end of the spectrum are the adenomas in FAP that are initiated by bi-allelic inactivation of APC. The phenotype associated with APC inactivation includes increased proliferation, crypt fission, and maturation arrest[109]. Many CRCs combine the phenotypic features that characterize the two ends of the polyp spectrum; that is, there may be evidence of inhibition of apoptosis and neo-expression of genes that characterize serrated polyps as well as the hyperproliferation and crypt division that are the hallmarks of adenomas. To put this differently, a serrated polyp could progress by acquiring adenomatous characteristics while an adenoma could progress by acquiring features of the serrated pathway. Thus while some CRC pathways may represent pure examples of the classical CIN and MSI-H models (with little or no overlap of genetic alterations) others, and perhaps the majority, may represent a fusion of the two classical routes of tumorigenesis (see 'third' pathway above).

An example of how this 'fusion' may occur has been described for the serrated pathway. *O-6-methylguanine DNA methyltransferase (MGMT)* removes pro-mutagenic adducts from guanine, and this direct DNA repair gene is silenced by methylation of its promoter region[110]. Loss of expression of MGMT has been shown by immunohistochemistry in serrated polyps[43,82]. Loss of expression of MGMT has been associated with C to T mutation in *TP53*[111]. Therefore, a pathway beginning with *BRAF* mutation and DNA methylation could, through loss of function of MGMT, acquire the features of the CIN pathway. Loss of expression of MGMT has also been linked to MSI-L[43,112] and to a type of chromosomal instability brought about by repeated or futile cycles of DNA excision and attempted repair at the site of methylG:T mismatches[113].

Loss of MGMT expression is not limited to serrated polyps but occurs also in adenomas, particularly villous adenomas[114]. Here, the failure to repair methylG:T mismatches may be associated with G to A mutation in *KRAS*[115], a gene that is closely linked with the initiation of serrated polyps. As noted above, there is frequent mutation of *APC*[20] and *KRAS*[30] in villous adenoma, and this lesion may represent a 'bridge' between the far more common tubular adenoma (with *APC* mutation) and hyperplastic polyp (with *KRAS* mutation) Therefore, inactivation of *MGMT* may serve as a 'cross-over' point between the two classical pathways and account for at least some 'fusion' pathways.

SUMMARY

There are cogent reasons to doubt the widely promulgated teaching that inactivation of the tumour-suppressor gene *APC* initiates most if not all adenomas, and furthermore that the 'vast majority' of CRCs arise within adenomas. While *APC* inactivation is always the initiating step in FAP adenomas this rule does not apply to all sporadic adenomas. It is also a fact that most adenomas are 'dead-end' lesions with little potential for further evolution. Some of the rare types of adenoma (villous, serrated, and flat), as well as variant hyperplastic polyps, may serve as the precursors of a relatively large proportion of CRCs. The reducing frequency of left-sided CRC with time may be partly explained by polypectomy but is not matched by a reducing frequency of right-sided CRCs[116]. Serrated polyps have been linked mainly with right-sided CRC. The lack of management guidelines for serrated polyps may be one explanation for the static incidence rates of right-sided CRC. In terms of chemoprevention, strategies that are targeted exclusively towards *APC* may not prevent the initiation of precancerous lesions of the colon that evolve through *APC*-independent pathways. By moving from the rigid and overly simplistic view of *APC* mutation as the first step in the evolution of virtually all CRCs, it is likely that progress in the prevention and early detection of this disease will occur rapidly.

References

1. Muto T, Bussey HJ, Morson BC. The evolution of cancer of the colon and rectum. Cancer. 1975;36:2251–70.
2. Vogelstein B, Fearon ER, Hamilton SR et al. Genetic alterations during colorectal-tumor development. N Engl J Med. 1988;319:525–32.
3. Konishi F, Morson BC. Pathology of colorectal adenomas: a colonoscopic survey. J Clin Pathol. 1982;35:830–41.
4. Jass JR, Young J, Leggett BA. Evolution of colorectal cancer: change of pace and change of direction. J Gastroenterol Hepatol. 2002;17:17–26.
5. Smith G, Carey FA, Beattie J et al. Mutations in APC, Kirsten-ras, and p53 - alternative genetic pathways to colorectal cancer. Proc Natl Acad Sci USA. 2002;99:9433–8.
6. Frattini D, Balestra D, Suardi S et al. Different genetic features associated with colon and rectal carcinogenesis. Clin Cancer Res. 2004;10:4015–21.
7. Fujiwara T, Stoker JM, Watanabe T et al. Accumulated clonal genetic alterations in familial and sporadic colorectal carcinomas with widespread instability in microsatellite sequences. Am J Pathol. 1998;153:1063–78.
8. Jass JR, Biden KG, Cummings M et al. Characterisation of a subtype of colorectal cancer combining features of the suppressor and mild mutator pathways. J Clin Pathol. 1999;52:455–60.
9. Simms LA, Radford-Smith G, Biden KG et al. Reciprocal relationship between the tumor suppressors p53 and BAX in primary colorectal cancers. Oncogene. 1998;17:2003–8.
10. Salahshor S, Kressner U, Påhlman L, Glimelius B, Lindmark G, Lindblom A. Colorectal cancer with and without microsatellite instability involves different genes. Genes Chromosomes Cancer. 1999;26:247–52.
11. Olschwang S, Hamelin R, Laurent-Puig P et al. Alternative genetic pathways in colorectal carcinogenesis. Proc Natl Acad Sci USA. 1997;94:12122–7.
12. Kambara T, Simms LA, Whitehall VLJ et al. BRAF mutation and CpG island methylation: an alternative pathway to colorectal cancer. Gut. 2004;53:1137–44.
13. Markowitz S, Wang J, Myeroff L et al. Inactivation of the type II TGF-β receptor in colon cancer cells with microsatellite instability. Science. 1995;268:1336–8.
14. Rampino N, Yamamoto H, Ionov Y et al. Somatic frameshift mutations in the *BAX* gene in colon cancers of the microsatellite mutator phenotype. Science. 1997;275:967–9.
15. Jen J, Powell SM, Papadopoulos N et al. Molecular determinants of dysplasia in colorectal lesions. Cancer Res. 1994;54:5523–6.
16. Takayama T, Ohi M, Hayashi T et al. Analysis of K-ras, APC, and beta-catenin in aberrant crypt foci in sporadic adenoma, cancer, and familial adenomatous polyposis. Gastroenterology. 2001;121:599–611.
17. Otori K, Konishi M, Sugiyama K et al. Infrequent somatic mutation of the adenomatous polyposis coli gene in aberrant crypt foci of human colon tissue. Cancer. 1998;83:896–900.
18. Umetani N, Sasaki S, Masaki T, Watanabe T, Matsuda K, Muto T. Involvement of APC and K-ras mutation in non-polypoid colorectal tumorigenesis. Br J Cancer. 2000;82:9–15.
19. Kim JC, Koo KH, Lee DH et al. Mutations at the APC exon 15 in the colorectal neoplastic tissues of serial array. Int J Colorectal Dis. 2001;16:102–7.
20. De Benedetti L, Sciallero S, Gismondi V et al. Association of APC gene mutations and histological characteristics of colorectal adenomas. Cancer Res. 1994;54:3553–6.
21. Mulkens J, Poncin J, Arends JW, De Goeij AF. APC mutations in human colorectal adenomas: analysis of the mutation cluster region with temperature gradient gel electrophoresis and clinicopathological features. J Pathol. 1998;185:360–5.

22. Zauber NP, Sabbath-Solitare M, Marotta SP, Bishop DT. K-ras mutation and loss of heterozygosity of the adenomatous polyposis coli gene in patients with colorectal adenomas with in situ carcinoma. Cancer. 1999;86:31–6.
23. Fodde R, Smits R, Clevers H. *APC*, signal transduction and genetic instability in colorectal cancer. Nature Rev Cancer. 2001;1:55–67.
24. Johnson V, Volikos E, Halford SER, et al. Exon 3 beta-catenin mutations are specifically associated with colorectal carcinomas in the hereditary non-polyposis colorectal cancer syndrome. Gut. 2004;53:264–7.
25. Esteller M, Sparks A, Toyota M et al. Analysis of adenomatous polyposis coli promoter hypermethylation in human cancer. Cancer Res. 2000;60:4366–71.
26. Liu W, Dong X, Mai M et al. Mutations in *AXIN2* cause colorectal cancer with defective mismatch repair by activating ß-catenin/TCF signalling. Nature Genet. 2000;26:146–7.
27. Thorstensen L, Lind GE, Lovig T et al. Genetic and epigenetic changes of components affecting the WNT pathway in colorectal carcinomas stratified by microsatellite instability. Neoplasia. 2005;7:99–108.
28. Janssen K-P, El Marjou F, Pinto D et al. Targetted expression of oncogenic K-ras in intestinal epithelium causes spontaneous tumorigenesis in mice. Gastroenterology. 2002; 123:492–504.
29. Li J, Mizukami Y, Zhang X, Jo W-S, Chung DC. Oncogenic K-ras stimulates Wnt signaling in colon cancer through inhibition of GSK-3beta. Gastroenterology. 2005;128:1907–18.
30. Maltzman T, Knoll K, Martinez ME et al. Ki-ras proto-oncogene mutations in sporadic colorectal adenomas: relationship to histologic and clinical characteristics. Gastroenterology. 2001;121:302–9.
31. Otori K, Oda Y, Sugiyama K et al. High frequency of K-*ras* mutations in human colorectal hyperplastic polyps. Gut. 1997;40:660–3.
32. Ajioka Y, Watanabe H, Jass JR, Yokota Y, Kobayashi M, Nishikura K. Infrequent K-ras codon 12 mutation in serrated adenomas of human colorectum. Gut. 1998;42:680–4.
33. Cox AD, Der CJ. The dark side of Ras: regulation of apoptosis. Oncogene. 2003;22:8999–9006.
34. Nascimbeni R, Villanacci V, Mariani PP et al. Aberrant crypt foci in the human colon. Am J Surg Pathol. 1999;23:1256–63.
35. Iino H, Jass JR, Simms LA et al. DNA microsatellite instability in hyperplastic polyps, serrated adenomas, and mixed polyps: a mild mutator pathway for colorectal cancer? J Clin Pathol. 1999;52:5–9.
36. Samowitz WS, Powers MD, Spirio LN, Nollet F, van Roy F, Slattery ML. ß-*Catenin* mutations are more frequent in small colorectal adenomas than in larger adenomas and invasive carcinomas. Cancer Res. 1999;59:1442–4.
37. Kinzler KW, Vogelstein B. Lessons from hereditary colorectal cancer. Cell. 1996;87:159–70.
38. Kane MF, Loda M, Gaida GM et al. Methylation of the hMLH1 promoter correlates with lack of expression of hMLH1 in sporadic colon tumors and mismatch repair-defective human tumor cell lines. Cancer Res. 1997;57:808–11.
39. Georgiades IB, Curtis LJ, Morris RM, Bird CC, Wyllie AH. Heterogeneity studies identify a subset of sporadic colorectal cancers without evidence for chromosomal or microsatellite instability. Oncogene. 1999;18:7933–40.
40. Hawkins NJ, Tomlinson I, Meagher A, Ward RL. Microsatellite-stable diploid carcinoma: a biologically distinct and aggressive subset of colorectal cancer. Br J Cancer. 2001;84:232–6.
41. Goel A, Arnold CN, Niedzwiecki D et al. Characterization of sporadic colon cancer by patterns of genomic instability. Cancer Res. 2003;63:1608–14.
42. Hawkins N, Norrie M, Cheong K et al. CpG island methylation in sporadic colorectal cancer and its relationship to microsatellite instability. Gastroenterology. 2002;122:1376–87.
43. Whitehall VLJ, Walsh MD, Young J, Leggett BA, Jass JR. Methylation of O-6-methylguanine DNA methyltransferase characterises a subset of colorectal cancer with low level DNA microsatellite instability. Cancer Res. 2001;61:827–30.
44. Whitehall VLJ, Wynter CVA, Walsh MD et al. Morphological and molecular heterogeneity within non-microsatellite instability-high colorectal cancer. Cancer Res. 2002;62:6011–14.

45. Young J, Barker MA, Simms LA et al. BRAF mutation and variable levels of microsatellite instability characterize a syndrome of familial colorectal cancer. Clin Gastroenterol Hepatol. 2005;3:254–63.
46. Rudzki Z, Zazula M, Okon K, Stachura J. Low-level microsatellite instability colorectal carcinomas: do they really belong to a 'gray zone' between high-level microsatellite instability and microsatellite-stable cancers? Int J Colorectal Dis. 2003;18:216–21.
47. Ward RL, Cheon K, Ku S-U, Meagher A, O'Connor T, Hawkins NJ. Adverse prognostic effect of methylation in colorectal cancer is reversed by microsatellite instability. J Clin Oncol. 2003;21:3729–36.
48. Tang R, C.R. C, Wu M-C et al. Colorectal cancer without high microsatellite instability and chromosomal instability – an alternative genetic pathway to human colorectal cancer. Carcinogenesis. 2004;25:841–6.
49. Yamashita K, Dai T, Dai Y, Yamamoto F, Perucho M. Genetics supersedes epigenetics in colon cancer phenotype. Cancer Cell. 2003;4:121–31.
50. Samowitz WS, Sweeney C, Herrick J et al. Poor survival associated with the BRAF V600E mutation in microsatellite-stable colon cancers. Cancer Res. 2005;65:6063–9.
51. Morson BC, Sobin LH. Histological Typing of Intestinal Tumours, 1st edn. Berlin: Springer-Verlag, 1976.
52. Spratt JS, Ackerman LV, Moyer CA. Relationships of polyps of the colon to colonic cancer. Ann Surg. 1958;148:682–96.
53. Bussey HJR. Familial Polyposis Coli. Baltimore: Johns Hopkins Press, 1975.
54. Eide TJ. Risk of colorectal cancer in adenoma-bearing individuals within a defined population. Int J Cancer. 1986;38:173–6.
55. Al-Tassan N, Chmiel NH, Maynard J et al. Inherited variants of MYH asociated with somatic G:C–T:A mutations in colorectal tumors. Nature Genet. 2002;30:227–32.
56. Kambara T, Whitehall VLJ, Spring KJ et al. Role of inherited defects of MYH in the development of sporadic colorectal cancer. Genes Chromosomes Cancer. 2004;40:1–9.
57. Almendingen K, Hofstad B, Vatn MH. Does a family history of cancer increase the risk of occurrence, growth, and recurrence of colorectal cancer. Gut. 2003;52:747–51.
58. Jass JR. Colorectal adenomas in surgical specimens from subjects with hereditary non-polyposis colorectal cancer. Histopathology. 1995;27:263–7.
59. Jass JR, Stewart SM. Evolution of hereditary non-polyposis colorectal cancer. Gut. 1992; 33:783–6.
60. Jass JR, Stewart SM, Stewart J, Lane MR. Hereditary non-polyposis colorectal cancer: morphologies, genes and mutations. Mutat Res. 1994;290:125–33.
61. de Jong AE, Morreau H, van Puijenbroek M et al. The role of mismatch repair gene defects in the development of adenomas in patients with HNPCC. Gastroenterology. 2004;126:42–8.
62. Vasen HFA, Nagengast FM, Meera Khan P. Interval cancers in hereditary non-polyposis colorectal cancer (Lynch syndrome). Lancet. 1995;345:1183–4.
63. Lynch HT, Smyrk T, Lynch JF. Overview of natural history, pathology, molecular genetics and mangement of HNPCC (Lynch syndrome). Int J Cancer. 1996;69:38–43.
64. Aaltonen LA, Peltomaki PS, Leach FS et al. Clues to the pathogenesis of familial colorectal cancer. Science. 1993;260:812–16.
65. Konishi M, Kikuchi-Yanoshita R, Tanaka K et al. Molecular nature of colon tumors in hereditary nonpolyposis colon cancer, familial polyposis, and sporadic colon cancer. Gastroenterology. 1996;111:307–17.
66. Huang J, Papadopoulos N, McKinley AJ et al. APC mutations in colorectal tumors with mismatch repair deficiency. Proc Natl Acad Sci USA. 1996;93:9049–54.
67. Miyaki M, Iijima T, Kimura J et al. Frequent mutation of β-catenin and APC genes in primary colorectal tumors from patients with hereditary nonpolyposis colorectal cancer. Cancer Res. 1999;59:4506–9.
68. Mirabelli-Primdahl L, Gryfe R, Kim H et al. Beta-catenin mutations are specific for colorectal carcinomas with microsatellite instability but occur in endometrial carcinomas irrespective of mutator pathway. Cancer Res. 1999;59:3346–51.
69. Akiyama Y, Nagasaki H, Yagi KO, Nomizu T, Yuasa Y. Beta-catenin and adenomatous polyposis coli (APC) mutations in adenomas from hereditary non-polyposis colorectal cancer patients. Cancer Lett. 2000;157:185–91.

70. Powell SM, Zilz N, Beazer-Barclay Y et al. APC mutations occur early during colorectal tumorigenesis. Nature. 1992;359:235–7.
71. Huang J, Zheng S, Jin S-H, Zhang S-Z. Somatic mutations of APC gene in carcinomas from hereditary non-polyposis colorectal cancer patients. World J Gastroenterol. 2004;10: 834–6.
72. Homfray TF, Cottrell SE, Ilyas M et al. Defects in mismatch repair occur after *APC* mutations in the pathogenesis of sporadic colorectal tumours. Hum Mutat. 1998;11:114–20.
73. Blank M, Klussmann E, Kruger-Krasagakes S et al. Expression of MUC2-mucin in colorectal adenomas and carcinomas of different histological types. Int J Cancer. 1994;59: 301–6.
74. Robertson DJ, Greenberg ER, Beach M et al. Colorectal cancer in patients under close colonoscopic surveillance. Gastroenterology. 2005;129:34–41.
75. Longacre TA, Fenoglio-Preiser CM. Mixed hyperplastic adenomatous polyps/serrated adenomas. A distinct form of colorectal neoplasia. Am J Surg Pathol. 1990;14:524–37.
76. Goldman H, Ming S, Hickock DF. Nature and significance of hyperplastic polyps of the human colon. Arch Pathol. 1970;89:349–54.
77. Biemer-Hüttmann A-E, Walsh MD, McGuckin MA et al. Immunohistochemical staining patterns of MUC1, MUC2, MUC4, and MUC5AC mucins in hyperplastic polyps, serrated adenomas, and traditional adenomas of the colorectum. J Histochem Cytochem. 1999;47: 1039–47.
78. Lazarus R, Junttila OE, Karttunen TJ, Makinen MJ. The risk of metachronous neoplasia in patients with serrated adenoma. Am J Clin Pathol. 2005;123:349–59.
79. Mäkinen MJ, George SMC, Jernvall P, Mäkelä J, Vihko P, Karttunen TJ. Colorectal carcinoma associated with serrated adenoma – prevalence, histological features, and prognosis. J Pathol. 2001;193:286–94.
80. Park S-J, Rashid A, Lee J-H, Kim SG, Hamilton SR, Wu TT. Frequent CpG island methylation in serrated adenomas of the colorectum. Am J Pathol. 2003;162:815–22.
81. Biemer-Hüttmann A-E, Walsh MD, McGuckin MA, Young J, Leggett BA, Jass JR. Mucin core protein expression in colorectal cancers with high levels of microsatellite instability indicates a novel pathway of morphogenesis. Clin Cancer Res. 2000;6:1909–16.
82. Sawyer EJ, Cerar A, Hanby AM et al. Molecular characteristics of serrated adenomas. Gut. 2002;51:200–6.
83. Jass JR, Young J, Leggett BA. Hyperplastic polyps and DNA microsatellite unstable cancers of the colorectum. Histopathology. 2000;37:295–301.
84. Jass JR, Iino H, Ruszkiewicz A et al. Neoplastic progression occurs through mutator pathways in hyperplastic polyposis of the colorectum. Gut. 2000;47:43–9.
85. Hawkins NJ, Ward RL. Sporadic colorectal cancers with microsatellite instability and their possible origin in hyperplastic polyps and serrated adenomas. J Natl Cancer Inst. 2001;93: 1307–13.
86. Torlakovic E, Skovlund E, Snover DC, Torlakovic G, Nesland JM. Morphologic reappraisal of serrated colorectal polyps. Am J Surg Pathol. 2003;27:65–81.
87. Goldstein NS, Bhanot P, Odish E, Hunter S. Hyperplastic-like colon polyps that preceded microsatellite unstable adenocarcinomas. Am J Clin Pathol. 2003;119:778–96.
88. Torlakovic E, Snover DC. Serrated adenomatous polyposis in humans. Gastroenterology. 1996;110:748–55.
89. O'Brien MJ, Yang S, Clebanoff JL et al. Hyperplastic (serrated) polyps of the colorectum. Relationship of CpG island methylator phenotype and K-ras mutation to location and histologic subtype. Am J Surg Pathol. 2004;28:423–34.
90. Wynter CVA, M.D. W, Higuchi T, Leggett BA, Young J, Jass JR. Methylation patterns define two types of hyperplastic polyp associated with colorectal cancer. Gut. 2004;53:573–80.
91. Batts KP. Serrated colorectal polyps: an update. Pathol Case Rev. 2004;9:173–82.
92. Higuchi T, Sugihara K, Jass JR. Demographic and pathological characteristics of serrated polyps of colorectum. Histopathology. 2005;47:32–40.
93. Jass JR. Hyperplastic-like polyps as precursors of microsatellite unstable colorectal cancer. Am J Clin Pathol. 2003;119:773—5.
94. Jass JR. Serrated adenoma of the colorectum and the DNA-methylator phenotype. Nat Clin Pract Oncol. 2005;2:398–405.

95. Yang S, Farraye FA, Mack C, Posnik O, O'Brien MJ. BRAF and KRAS mutations in hyperplastic polyps and serrated adenomas of the colorectum: relationship to histology and CpG island methylation status. Am J Surg Pathol. 2004;28:1452–9.
96. Spratt JSJ, Ackerman LV. Small primary adenocarcinomas of the colon and rectum. J Am Med Assoc. 1962;179:337–46.
97. Stolte M, Bethke B. Colorectal mini-*de novo* carcinoma: a reality in Germany too. Endoscopy. 1995;27:286–90.
98. Shimoda T, Ikegami M, Fujisaki J, Matsui T, Aizawa S, Ishikawa E. Early colorectal carcinoma with special reference to its development *de novo*. Cancer. 1989;64:1138–46.
99. Bedenne L, Faivre J, Boutron MC, Piard F, Cauvin JM, Hillon P. Adenoma–carcinoma sequence or '*de novo*' carcinogenesis? Cancer. 1992;69:883–8.
100. Muto T, Kamiya J, Sawada T et al. Small 'flat adenoma' of the large bowel with special reference to its clinicopathologic features. Dis Colon Rectum. 1985;28:847–51.
101. Kuramoto S, Oohara T. Minute cancers arising de novo in the human large intestine. Cancer. 1988;61:829–34.
102. Hart AR, Kudo S, Mackay EH, Mayberry JF, Atkin WS. Flat adenomas exist in asymptomatic people: important implications for colorectal cancer screening programmes. Gut. 1998;43:229–331.
103. Jaramillo E, Watanabe M, Slezak P, Rubio C. Flat neoplastic lesions of the colon and rectum detected by high-resolution video endoscopy and chromoscopy. Gastrointest Endosc. 1995;42:114–22.
104. Rembacken BJ, Fujii T, Cairns A et al. Flat and depressed colonic neoplasms: a prospective study of 1000 colonoscopies in the UK. Lancet. 2000;355:1211–14.
105. Saitoh Y, Waxman I, West AB et al. Prevalence and distinctive biologic features of flat colorectal adenomas in a North American population. Gastroenterology. 2001;120:1657–65.
106. Yamagata S, Muto T, Uchida Y et al. Lower incidence of K-*ras* codon 12 mutation in flat colorectal adenomas than in polypoid adenomas. Jpn J Cancer Res. 1994;85:147–51.
107. Nosho K, Yamamoto H, Adachi Y, Endo T, Hinoda Y, Imai K. Gene expression profiling of colorectal adenomas and early invasive carcinomas by cDNA array analysis. Br J Cancer. 2005;92:1193–200.
108. Jass JR. Hyperplastic polyps and colorectal cancer: Is there a link? Clin Gastroenterol Hepatol. 2004;2:1–8.
109. Wasan HS, Park H-S, Liu KC et al. APC in the regulation of intestinal crypt fission. J Pathol. 1998;185:246–55.
110. Esteller M, Hamilton SR, Burger PC, Baylin SB, Herman JG. Inactivation of the DNA repair gene O^6-*methylguanine-DNA methyltransferase* by promoter hypermethylation is a common event in primary human neoplasia. Cancer Res. 1999;59:793–7.
111. Esteller M, Risques RA, Toyota M et al. Promoter hypermethylation of the DNA repair gene O^6-*methylguanine-DNA methyltransferase* is associated with the presence of G:C to A:T transition mutations in *p53* in human colorectal tumorigenesis. Cancer Res. 2001;61:4689–92.
112. Kohonen-Corish MRJ, Daniel JJ, Chan C et al. Low microsatellite instability is associated with poor prognosis in stage C colon cancer. J Clin Oncol. 2005;23:2318–24.
113. Karran P, Bignami M. DNA damage tolerance, mismatch repair and genome instability. Bioessays. 1994;16:833–9.
114. Rashid A, Shen L, Morris JS, Issa J-PJ, Hamilton SR. CpG island methylation in colorectal adenomas. Am J Pathol. 2001;159:1129–35.
115. Esteller M, Toyota M, Sanchez-Cespedes M et al. Inactivation of the DNA repair gene O6-*methylguanine-DNA methyltransferase* by promoter hypermethylation is associated with G to A mutations in *K-ras* in colorectal tumorigenesis. Cancer Res. 2000;60:2368–71.
116. Rabeneck L, Davila JA, El-Serag HB. Is there a true 'shift' to the right colon in the incidence of colorectal cancer? Am J Gastroenterol. 2003;98:1400–9.

8
The molecular regulation of the malignant progression of human colorectal cancer

A. JUNG

INTRODUCTION

Colorectal cancer (CRC) is one of the human neoplasias with the highest morbidity. The development of CRC follows an adenoma–carcinoma sequence. The different stages in this sequence are easy to distinguish histologically. Moreover, CRC accumulate a variety of mutations in oncogenes (gain of function) such as K-ras and tumour-suppressor genes (loss of function) such as APC (adenomatous polyposis coli), p53 (the guardian of DNA), DCC (deleted in colorectal cancer) as well as members of the TGF-β (transforming growth factor β) pathway such as SMAD4 (mothers against decapentaplegic)/DPC4 (deleted in pancreatic carcinoma)[1]. This connection is known as the 'multistep carcinogenesis model' which has become a paradigm of carcinogenesis for all kind of tumours[2]. Moreover, there is no strict order in the appearance of mutations but usually APC is mutated very early in this process. Thus, APC is known as the gatekeeper of colorectal carcinogenesis[2]. APC is a central element in the Wnt signalling pathway[1]. Here it is an integral part of a degradation complex which is composed at least of axin/conductin, APC and GSK-3β (glycogen synthase kinse-3β)[1–3]. This complex plays a central role in the regulation of the stability of β-catenin, the executor of the Wnt-signalling pathway[3]. After binding to the degradation complex β-catenin is phosphorylated by GSK-3β, which is an earmark for the ubiquitination of β-catenin and the subsequent degradation by the 28S proteasome[1–4]. The activity of the degradation complex is regulated by Wnt-signalling. After a Wnt ligand binds to its receptors, members of the frizzled family which belong to the super-family of seven membrane spanning proteins[3], the degradation complex is muted by a not-completely-understood mechanism. Consequently β-catenin accumulates in the cytoplasm of affected cells. If APC is mutated the β-catenin degradation complex is inactive and thus β-catenin is not degraded any more – or at least at a very low frequency[1,2,4].

β-Catenin has a dual function. On the one hand it is an integral part of the zonula adhaerens. Here it bridges the cytoplasmic part of E-cadherin via α-catenin with the cell's cytoskeleton. By doing so it stabilizes the epithelial phenotype of affected cells[5]. If β-catenin has translocated into the nucleus of cells it works on the other hand as a transcription factor by interacting with members of the TCF (T-cell factor)/LEF-1 (lymphocyte-enhancing factor) family[6]. Dimers of β-catenin/(TCF/LEF-1) bind to the DNA and trans-activate gene expression of a variety of genes which are involved in several cellular processes such as migration, invasion, dissemination, growth control, apoptosis and other more[4], the typical hallmarks of cancer[7]. Moreover, nuclear β-catenin induces a mesenchymal phenotype[8]. This is achieved by the suppression of the E-cadherin gene expression via the up-regulation of inhibitors of E-cadherin gene expression such as members of the SNAI/ZEB family (slug)[9]. Thus, β-catenin is a central player in the regulation of epithelial to mesenchymal transition (EMT) depending on its subcellular localization[10].

According to the multistep carcinogenesis model the accumulation of gene mutations drives the malignant progression of colorectal tumours[2]. Malignant progression is accompanied by a gain in proliferation, the loss of epithelial differentiation and thus a gain in migration, invasion, and dissemination. This change can be nicely explained by the loss of function of the APC containing β-catenin degradation complex and the subsequent increase of nuclear β-catenin which drives mesenchymal transition by an alteration of the gene expression profile. On the other hand one would consequently expect that metastases of CRC should appear as an accumulation of cells which have lost their epithelial differentiation (dedifferentiation); but this is not the case[11]. Primary CRC, as well as their metastases, appear mostly well differentiated; moreover, β-catenin is found mainly at the cytoplasm-membrane in conjunction with E-cadherin[11,12]. The question then arises as to how CRC can metastasize at all? Histologically primary colorectal tumours, as well as the corresponding metastases, contain well-differentiated tumour cells with an epithelial phenotype in the central areas of the tumour. On the other hand tumour cells mostly found at the invasion front have lost their differentiation and appear mesenchymally organized[11,12]. This change in histological appearance is accompanied by a different subcellular localization of β-catenin. In well-differentiated tumour cells β-catenin is found together with E-cadherin at the membrane of the tumour cells[11]. In a dedifferentiated zone β-catenin is found in the nucleus[11]. Moreover, a variety of target genes are expressed in these cells, such as the extracellular matrix degrading proteases uPA (urokinase plasminogen activator)[13], MMP-7 (matrix metalloproteinase 7)[14], MT1-MMP (membrane type 1 matrix metalloproteinase)[15], or inducers of migration such as laminin-5γ 2[16] or TnC (tenascin-C)[17]. As these changes in the phenotype of the tumour cells are found in the primary tumours as well as in metastases they cannot be genetically fixed, if mutations are irreversibly fixed in the genome. Thus these phenotypical changes must be regulatable[11,18,19]. The driving force for the induction of the translocation of β-catenin might be contributed by the extracellular matrix or the environment of the tumour cells. Components of the extracellular matrix such as collagen I are able to induce changes in the differentiation of colorectal tumour cells in cell culture[20]. Moreover, nuclear localization of β-catenin and a down-regulation of E-cadherin are found after activation of ILK (integrin linked kinase)[18]. This kinase is linked to the intracellular domain of integrin dimers and is activated after interaction of integrins with their extracellular matrix components. Moreover, dedifferentiation is also seen together with scattering of tumour cells after encountering HGF (hepatocyte growth factor)[8,21], which is also a compound of the extracellular matrix. Finally, TGF-β (transforming growth factor β) is also known to be an inductor of EMT.

Taken together, a model of non-linear tumour progression might be postulated on these data. In this model the mutations found in CRC give colorectal tumour cells the capability for malignant growth. But malignant growth is regulated reversibly by the tumour environment by altering the subcellular localization of β-catenin. Thus, the histological heterogeneity of the tumours is reflected by a functional heterogeneity. Interestingly, the histological heterogeneity correlates highly significant with the 5-year survival of patients[32], which is further support for the relevance of the EMT found in CRC.

What might be the underlying mechanism in the tumour cells which is responsible for the different behaviour of the tumour cells, and which is reflected in an epithelial or mesenchymal differentiation? One possible and attractive view is that mesenchymally differentiated tumour cells characterized by nuclear β-catenin might be tumour stem cells. Several reasons support this view. First, normal adult stem cells express β-catenin in their nuclei as well in humans[23] as in the mouse[24]. Secondly, β-catenin target genes are indicative for stem cells. Thus, survivin is a β-catenin target gene[25,26] and is expressed in adult stem cells[27]. Another gene indicating stem cells or stemness is hTERT (human telomerase RT-component)[28], which is also under the control of β-catenin[29]. Thirdly, dedifferentiated colorectal tumour cells display low proliferation[30] as do stem cells in general[28]. This observation is at first glance contradictary as cells with nuclear β-catenin also express the β-catenin target genes c-myc[31] and directly or indirectly cyclin D_1[32–34]. The low proliferating activity is conferred by the expression of the cell cycle inhibitor p16[INL4a] (see ref. 21). Again, p16[INK4a] is a β-catenin target gene[35].

In such a case the biologically active component of human CRC would be represented by the small ridge of tumour cells at the invasion front of the tumours. But some tumour stem cells, indicated by the expression of survivin[27] are also found distributed in differentiated areas of the tumours found mainly in the central areas of the CRC.

References

1. Bienz M, Clevers H. Linking colorectal cancer to Wnt signaling. Cell. 2000;103:311–20.
2. Kinzler KW, Vogelstein B. Lessons from hereditary colorectal cancer. Cell. 1996;87:159–70.
3. Huelsken J, Behrens J. The Wnt signalling pathway. J Cell Sci. 2002;115:3977–8.
4. Brabletz T, Herrmann K, Jung A, Faller G, Kirchner T. Expression of nuclear β-catenin and c-myc is correlated with tumor size but not with proliferative activity of colorectal adenomas. Am J Pathol. 2000;156:865–70.
5. Nelson WJ, Nusse R. Convergence of Wnt, β-catenin, and cadherin pathways. Science. 2004;303:1483–7.

6. Lustig B, Behrens J. The Wnt signaling pathway and its role in tumor development. J Cancer Res Clin Oncol. 2003;129:199–221.
7. Hanahan D, Weinberg RA. The hallmarks of cancer. Cell. 2000;100:57–70.
8. Brembeck FH, Schwarz-Romond T, Bakkers J, Wilhelm S, Hammerschmidt M, Birchmeier W. Essential role of BCL9-2 in the switch between β catenin's adhesive and transcriptional functions. Genes Dev. 2004;18:2225–30.
9. Conacci-Sorrell M, Simcha I, Ben-Yedidia T, Blechman J, Savagner P, Ben-Ze'ev A. Autoregulation of E-cadherin expression by cadherin–cadherin interactions: the roles of β-catenin signaling, Slug, and MAPK. J Cell Biol. 2003;163:847–57.
10. Thiery JP. Epithelial-mesenchymal transitions in tumour progression. Nat Rev Cancer. 2002;2:442–54.
11. Brabletz T, Jung A, Reu S et al. Variable β-catenin expression in colorectal cancers indicates tumor progression driven by the tumor environment. Proc Natl Acad Sci USA. 2001;98: 10356–61.
12. Brabletz T, Jung A, Hermann K, Gunther K, Hohenberger W, Kirchner T. Nuclear overexpression of the oncoprotein β-catenin in colorectal cancer is localized predominantly at the invasion front. Pathol Res Pract. 1998;194:701–4.
13. Hiendlmeyer E, Regus S, Wassermann S et al. β-Catenin up-regulates the expression of the urokinase plasminogen activator in human colorectal tumors. Cancer Res. 2004;64:1209–14.
14. Brabletz T, Jung A, Dag S, Hlubek F, Kirchner T. β-Catenin regulates the expression of the matrix metalloproteinase-7 in human colorectal cancer. Am J Pathol. 1999;155:1033–8.
15. Hlubek F, Spaderna S, Jung A, Kirchner T, Brabletz T. β-Catenin activates a coordinated expression of the proinvasive factors laminin-5 γ2 chain and MT1-MMP in colorectal carcinomas. Int J Cancer. 2004;108:321–6.
16. Hlubek F, Jung A, Kotzor N, Kirchner T, Brabletz T. Expression of the invasion factor laminin γ2 in colorectal carcinomas is regulated by β-catenin. Cancer Res. 2001;61:8089–93.
17. Beiter K, Hiendlmeyer E, Brabletz T et al. β-Catenin regulates the expression of tenascin-C in human colorectal tumors. Oncogene. 2005;24:8200–4.
18. Barker N, Clevers H. Tumor environment: a potent driving force in colorectal cancer? Trends Mol Med. 2001;7:535–7.
19. Brabletz T, Jung A, Kirchner T. β-Catenin and the morphogenesis of colorectal cancer. Virchows Arch. 2002;441:1–11.
20. Brabletz T, Spaderna S, Kolb J et al. Down-regulation of the homeodomain factor Cdx2 in colorectal cancer by collagen type I: an active role for the tumor environment in malignant tumor progression. Cancer Res. 2004;64:6973–7.
21. Birchmeier C, Birchmeier W, Gherardi E, Vande Woude GF. Met, metastasis, motility and more. Nat Rev Mol Cell Biol. 2003;4:915–25.
22. Ueno H, Murphy J, Jass JR, Mochizuki H, Talbot IC. Tumour 'budding' as an index to estimate the potential of aggressiveness in rectal cancer. Histopathology. 2002;40:127–32.
23. Potten CS, Booth C, Tudor GL et al. Identification of a putative intestinal stem cell and early lineage marker; musashi-1. Differentiation. 2003;71:28–41.
24. van de Wetering M, Sancho E, Verweij C et al. The β-catenin/TCF-4 complex imposes a crypt progenitor phenotype on colorectal cancer cells. Cell. 2002;111:241–50.
25. Kim PJ, Plescia J, Clevers H, Fearon ER, Altieri DC. Survivin and molecular pathogenesis of colorectal cancer. Lancet. 2003;362:205–9.
26. Zhang T, Otevrel T, Gao Z, Ehrlich SM, Fields JZ, Boman BM. Evidence that APC regulates survivin expression: a possible mechanism contributing to the stem cell origin of colon cancer. Cancer Res. 2001;61:8664–7.
27. Brabletz T, Jung A, Hlubek F, Spaderna S, Kirchner T. Migrating tumor stem cells in colorectal cancer. Nat Rev Cancer. 2005;9:744–9.
28. Melton DA, Cowan C. Stemness: definitions, criteria and standards. In: Lanza R, editor. Essentials of Stem Cell Biology. Amsterdam: Elsevier, 2006: xxv–xxxi.
29. Hiendlmeyer E, Brabletz T, Haynl A, Herbst H, Kirchner T, Jung A. β-Catenin transactivates the expression of hTERT (human telomerase RT-component) in colorectal tumors indicating thereby tumor stem cells (Under revision).

30. Jung A, Schrauder M, Oswald U et al. The invasion front of human colorectal adenocarcinomas shows co- localization of nuclear β-catenin, cyclin D1, and p16INK4A and is a region of low proliferation. Am J Pathol. 2001;159:1613–17.
31. He TC, Sparks AB, Rago C et al. Identification of c-MYC as a target of the APC pathway. Science. 1998;281:1509–12.
32. Sansom OJ, Reed KR, van de Wetering M et al. Cyclin D1 is not an immediate target of β-catenin following Apc loss in the intestine. J Biol Chem. 2005;280:28463–7.
33. Shtutman M, Zhurinsky J, Simcha I et al. The cyclin D1 gene is a target of the β-catenin/ LEF-1 pathway. Proc Natl Acad Sci USA. 1999;96:5522–7.
34. Tetsu O, McCormick F. β-Catenin regulates expression of cyclin D1 in colon carcinoma cells. Nature. 1999;398:422–6.
35. Wassermann S, Hiendlmeyer E, Palmqvist R et al. The cell cycle-inhibitor p16[INK4a] is regulated by β-catenin and predicts survival in human colorectal cancer (Submitted) (2006).

Section IV
Colorectal cancer: new screening strategies for the new millenium

Chair: M.M. LERCH and M. ZEITZ

9
Impact of the National Polyp Study

S. J. WINAWER

BACKGROUND AND GOALS OF THE NATIONAL POLYP STUDY (NPS)

Colorectal cancer screening came into generalized clinical use in the early 1970s with the introduction of guaiac card faecal occult blood tests, flexible sigmoidoscopy and colonoscopy, and the demonstration of the feasibility of removing polyps through colonoscopy[1]. Earlier attempts at colorectal cancer screening were based on bench guaiac reagents or benzidine and the barium enema. The new 1970s technology provided a package of more sensitive and specific standardized stool tests, accurate diagnosis with colonoscopy and effective treatment by colonoscopic polypectomy and cancer resection based on modern surgical concepts.

It soon became clear that the adenomatous polyp was by far the more common neoplastic lesion detected by screening, and that there were no guidelines as to how to follow these patients in order to reduce their risk of cancer. A joint research committee was organized in 1978 by the American Gastroenterology Association, the American Society of Gastrointestinal Endoscopy, later joined by the American College of Gastroenterology to develop a protocol with, as its major objective, the evaluation of strategies for the surveillance of patients after polypectomy to control large bowel cancer. It was decided that a randomized prospective trial was needed to provide data on which to base guidelines for follow-up surveillance of these patients (Table 1). At the time different intervals and methods of follow-up were being used, and when colonoscopy was the method of choice it was usually performed annually after polypectomy[2].

Although the major objective of the NPS was to provide data on follow-up surveillance, the study could also provide the opportunity to learn more about the natural history of the colonic adenoma and its relationship to colorectal cancer. Although the adenoma–carcinoma progression was widely accepted, there was no evidence that removal of adenomas would reduce the risk of colorectal cancer[1]. In addition, the NPS could provide data regarding the effectiveness in surveillance of the faecal occult blood test and double-contrast barium enema relative to colonoscopy, the importance of predictors of subsequent adenomas especially familial factors, other pathological findings including hyperplastic polyps and flat adenomas[2].

Table 1 National Polyp Study

Randomized trial
Surveillance intervals
Surveillance methods
CRC incidence
Adenoma–carcinoma model
Seven clinical centres
MSK coordinating centre

DESIGN OF THE NPS: ELIGIBILITY

All patients referred for initial colonoscopy or polypectomy at seven participating centres who did not have a family or personal history of familial polyposis, inflammatory bowel disease, or a personal history of polypectomy or colorectal cancer were identified prospectively from November 1980 through February 1990. Patients were excluded if colonoscopy revealed colorectal cancer, non-adenomatous polyps, malignant polyps (adenomas with cancer invading beyond the muscularis mucosa), and a sessile adenoma with a base larger than 3 cm, or the absence of polyps. Patients were eligible if they underwent a complete colonoscopy to the level of the caecum, with removal of all polyps detected, and were found to have one or more adenomas. The study protocol was approved annually by the institutional review board of each participating centre. The following information was ascertained for all patients: reason for referral, age and sex, and the presence or absence of a family history of colorectal cancer, a personal history of other cancers, and polyps in first-degree relatives[2].

DESIGN: STRATIFICATION, RANDOMIZATION, AND FOLLOW-UP

Eligible patients consenting to enroll in the study were stratified according to the study centre, the number of adenomas (single or multiple), and the histological type of adenoma (tubular or villous). The patients were randomly assigned within the appropriate stratum to have a follow-up examination either 1 and 3 years after colonoscopy (the two-examination group) or 3 years after colonoscopy (the one-examination group). (A follow-up colonoscopy 6 years after the examination at entry was also offered to both groups.) Blocked randomization within strata was used to ensure balance between the two groups over time. The study coordinator contacted all patients annually to complete an interval-history questionnaire and to schedule colonoscopies[2].

Endoscopy and pathological review

All endoscopic examinations were performed by study investigators. Each polyp removed was placed in a bottle, labelled according to the anatomical segment involved (caecum, ascending colon, hepatic flexure, transverse colon, splenic flexure, descending colon, sigmoid, or rectum), and classified as sessile or pedunculated. The size of the polyp before polypectomy was estimated with use of open biopsy forceps, and the method of removal (i.e. biopsy fulguration or cautery snare) was recorded. Polyps were classified as small (<0.5 cm in diameter), medium (0.6–1.0 cm), or large (>1.0 cm). Serial sections of each polyp were obtained from the participating institutions and coded consecutively on an individual case basis for simultaneous examination at a multihead microscope by the three review pathologists according to uniform criteria established at the beginning of the study; a consensus was reached about each polyp without knowledge of the clinical data or the study centre from which it came. The number of sections varied according to the size of the polyp. Additional sections were obtained if high-grade dysplasia or invasive cancer was present. Adenomas were classified as tubular or villous. Villous adenomas were classified according to the proportion of villous component: class A, 1–25%; class B, 26–75%; class C, 76–99%; and class D, 100%. All reports were based on the classification of the polyps after pathological review. An adenoma was defined as having advanced pathological features if it was large (>1.0 cm) or had high-grade dysplasia or invasive cancer[3].

STATISTICAL ANALYSIS

A total enrollment of 1400 patients was planned, under the assumption that 975 patients would survive and undergo a follow-up colonoscopy within the study period. The study was designed to detect a difference in the percentage of patients who had adenomas with advanced pathological features detected at 1 year of 3% (the two-examination group), in comparison to 7% at 3 years (the one-examination group), with a power of 80% and a level of significance of 0.05 (two-sided); the difference between percentages was equivalent to a relative risk of 2.3 or more. The relative risk that any adenomas, as well as adenomas with advanced pathological features would be detected at follow-up 3 years after entry colonoscopy (the one-examination group) as compared with only 1 year (the two-examination group) was calculated along with a 95% confidence interval. Logistic regression was used to assess the odds of detecting adenomas with advanced pathological features at 3 years as compared with 1 year, with control for the stratification variables of the histological type of adenoma, number of adenomas, and study centre. In addition, logistic regression was used to assess independent risk factors for adenomas with advanced pathological features detected at the first follow-up examination and to examine the effects of any interaction between study-group assignment and characteristics at enrollment. The likelihood-ratio test was used to determine whether a variable was an independent risk factor for the detection of adenomas with advanced pathological features[2].

Similar analyses were performed with respect to adenomas with advanced pathological features detected at the second follow-up examination in the two-examination group as compared with those detected at follow-up in the one-examination group. The percentage of patients who had adenomas with advanced pathological features detected at either follow-up examination in the two-examination group was compared with the percentage with such adenomas in the one-examination group. The Wilcoxon test was used to determine whether the number of adenomas detected at follow-up differed in the two groups. All *p* values were two-sided; all analyses were performed with SAS and BMDP software packages[4–7].

RESULTS OF NPS STUDIES
Randomized comparison of surveillance intervals after colonoscopic removal of newly diagnosed adenomatous polyps[8]

Of 2632 eligible patients, 1418 were randomly assigned to the two follow-up groups, 699 to the two-examination group and 719 to the one-examination group. The proportion of patients with adenomas in the group examined at 1 and 3 years was 41.7%, as compared with 32.0% in the group examined at 3 years (*p* = 0.006). The proportion of patients with adenomas with advanced pathological features was the same in both groups (3.3%) (Figure 1). Colonoscopy performed 3 years after colonoscopic removal of adenomatous polyps therefore detected important colonic lesions as effectively as follow-up colonoscopy after both 1 and 3 years. An interval of at least three years was therefore recommended before follow-up examination after colonoscopic removal of newly diagnosed adenomatous polyps. Adoption of this recommendation nationally should reduce the cost of post-polypectomy surveillance and screening.

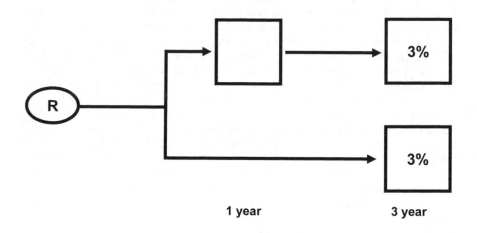

Figure 1   National Polyp Study. Advanced adenomas at follow-up[8] (See text for details and explanation)

Prevention of colorectal cancer by colonoscopic polypectomy[9]

The study cohort consisted of 1418 patients who had a complete colonoscopy during which one or more adenomas of the colon or rectum were removed. The patients subsequently underwent periodic colonoscopy during an average follow-up of 5.9 years, and the incidence of colorectal cancer was ascertained. The incidence rate of colorectal cancer was compared with that in three reference groups, including two cohorts in which colonic polyps were not removed and one general-population registry (SEER), after adjustment for sex, age, and polyp size. Ninety-seven per cent of the patients were followed clinically for a total of 8401 person-years, and 80% returned for one or more of their scheduled colonoscopies. Five asymptomatic early-stage colorectal cancers (malignant polyps) were detected by colonoscopy (three at 3 years, one at 6 years, and one at 7 years). No symptomatic cancers were detected. The numbers of colorectal cancers expected on the basis of the rates in the three reference groups were 48.3, 43.4, and 20.7, for reductions in the incidence of colorectal cancer of 90%, 88%, and 76%, respectively ($p < 0.001$) (Figure 2). Colonoscopic polypectomy resulted in a lower-than-expected incidence of colorectal cancer. These results supported the view that colorectal adenomas progress to adenocarcinomas, as well as the current practice of searching for and removing adenomatous polyps to prevent colorectal cancer.

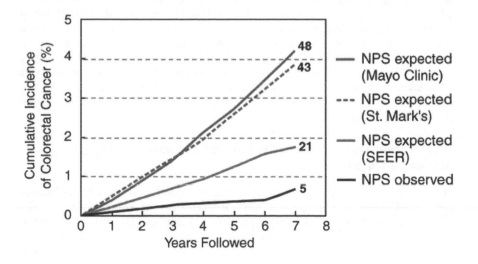

Figure 2 Colorectal cancer incidence in NPS following colonoscopy polypectomy (1418 patients; 8401 person-years)[9] (See text for details and explanation)

A comparison of colonoscopy and double-contrast barium enema for surveillance after polypectomy[10]

After patients have undergone colonoscopic polypectomy, it is uncertain whether colonoscopic examination or a barium enema was the better method of surveillance. As part of the National Polyp Study we offered both colonoscopic examination and double-contrast barium enema for surveillance to patients with newly diagnosed adenomatous polyps. Although barium enema was performed first, the endoscopist did not know the results. A blinded and unblinded colonoscopy method was developed in relation to a previously performed barium enema for an unbiased comparison that would not compromise patient risk. A total of 973 patients underwent one or more colonoscopic examinations for surveillance. In the case of 580 of these patients we performed 862 paired colonoscopic examinations and barium enema examinations that met the requirements of the protocol. The findings on barium enema were positive in 222 (26%) of the paired examinations, including 94 of the 242 colonoscopic examinations in which one or more adenomas were detected (rate of detection of adenomas, 39%; 95% confidence interval (CI), 33–45%). The proportion of examinations in which adenomatous polyps were detected by barium enema was significantly related to the size of the adenomas ($p = 0.009$); the rate was 32% for colonoscopic examinations in which the largest adenomas detected were 0.5 cm or less, 53% for those in which the largest adenomas detected were 0.6–1.0 cm, and 48% for those in which the largest adenomas detected exceeded 1.0 cm. Among the 139 paired examinations with positive results on barium enema and negative results on colonoscopic examination in the same location, 19 additional polyps, 12 of which were adenomas, were detected on colonoscopic re-examination. We concluded that, in patients who have undergone colonoscopic polypectomy, colonoscopic examination is a more effective method of surveillance than double-contrast barium enema.

Risk of colorectal cancer in the families of patients with adenomatous polyps[11]

A random sample of participants in the National Polyp Study who had newly diagnosed adenomatous polyps were interviewed for information on the history of colorectal cancer in their parents and siblings. The risk of colorectal cancer in family members was analysed according to the characteristics of the patients with adenomas and in comparison with a sample of patients' spouses, who served as controls. Among the patients with adenomas, 1199 provided information on whether they had a family history of colorectal cancer. After the exclusion of families for which information was incomplete, and of 48 patients who had been referred for colonoscopy solely because they had a family history of colorectal cancer, there were 1031 patients with adenomas, 1865 parents, 2381 siblings, and 1411 spouse controls. The relative risk of colorectal cancer, adjusted for the year of birth and sex, was 1.78 for the parents and siblings of the patients with adenomas as compared with the spouse controls (95% CI 1.18–2.67). The relative risk for siblings of patients in whom adenomas were diagnosed before 60 years of age was 2.59 (95% CI 1.46–4.58), as compared with the siblings of patients who were 60 or older at the time of diagnosis and after adjustment for the sibling's year of birth and sex and a parental history of colorectal cancer. The risk increased with decreasing age at the time of the diagnosis of adenoma (p for trend <0.001). The relative risk for the siblings of patients who had a parent with colorectal cancer, as compared with those who had no parent with cancer, was 3.25 (95% CI 1.92–5.52), after adjustment for the sibling's year of birth and sex and the patient's age at diagnosis. Siblings and parents of patients with adenomatous polyps are at increased risk for colorectal cancer, particularly when the adenoma is diagnosed before the age of 60 or – in the case of siblings – when a parent has had colorectal cancer.

Can surveillance intervals be lengthened following colonoscopic polypectomy?[12]

Among the 1418 patients who underwent randomization because of the presence of one or more adenomas and with no exclusion criteria, 522 had follow-up colonoscopies at 1, 3 and 6 years in arm A and 416 had follow-up colonoscopies at 3 and 6 years in arm B. The baseline characteristics were the same in both arms in terms of demographics and polyp characteristics as previously reported. (NPS 1993) Over the follow-up surveillance period of 6 years there were the same number of adenomas with advanced pathology in arm A and arm B. Baseline characteristics were examined in a multivariant analysis to determine predictors of advanced pathology at follow-up surveillance over the 6-year period. The relative risk for advanced adenomas was 2.7 (CI 1.31–5.75) for patients equal to or over age 60 as compared to patients under age 60 (Figure). The relative risk was 2.02 (CI 1.03–4.81) for patients equal to or greater than age 60 and a negative parenteral history of colorectal cancer and 6.06 (CI 2.45–14.95) for patients equal to or greater than age 60 with a positive parental history of colorectal cancer as compared to patients under age 60. The relative risk of males was 1.5 (CI 0.60–2.21) compared to females. The relative risk for advanced adenomas for patients with adenomas 0.6–1.0 cm was 1.3 (CI 0.47–3.92) and 2.91 for patients with adenomas >1.0 cm (CI 1.12–7.59) compared to patients with adenomas equal to or less than 0.5 cm at baseline. There was an increased relative risk for advanced pathology at surveillance for patients with more advanced pathology at baseline. The relative risk for adenomas with advanced pathology at surveillance for patients with two adenomas at baseline was 1.80 (CI 0.70–4.65); and 6.11 (CI 2.99–12.48) for patients with three or more adenomas at baseline. Patients were stratified into two groups: those at low risk for adenomas at surveillance and those at higher risk for adenomas at surveillance over the 6-year follow-up based on baseline characteristics. Low-risk patients were those with less than two adenomas and age >60 with a negative family history of colorectal cancer; and high-risk patients were those with three or more adenomas and age >60 with a positive family history of colorectal cancer. The high-risk patients had a relative risk of advanced adenomas of 6.24 (CI 3.25–12.02) compared to the low-risk patients.

Flat adenomas in the National Polyp Study: is there increased risk for high-grade dysplasia initially or during surveillance[13]?

The flat adenoma may be a more aggressive pathway in colorectal carcinogenesis. Sessile adenomas from the National Polyp Study cohort were reclassified histopathologically as flat or polypoid using an optical and microscopic measuring device and correlated in a blinded comparison with initial and surveillance pathology. A total of 933 sessile adenomas detected during 1980–1990 were reclassified as follows: (1) adenoma thickness (AT): < 1.3 mm, and (2) adenoma ratio (AR): adenoma thickness $< 2 \times$ normal mucosa thickness. Logistic regression was used to assess whether flat adenomas had an effect on risk for high-grade dysplasia initially, and a Cox proportional hazards model assessed the risk for advanced adenomas at surveillance. The analysis encompassed 8401 person-years of follow-up evaluation. AT and AR measures of adenoma flatness were 95% concordant. By the AT measure, flat adenomas ($n = 474$) represented 27% of all baseline adenomas. Flat adenomas were found to be no more likely to exhibit high-grade dysplasia than sessile (polypoid) or pedunculated adenomas, the odds ratio for high-grade dysplasia was 1.91 (95% CI 0.66–5.47; $p = 0.23$) for sessile (polypoid) vs flat adenomas and 1.78 (95% CI 0.63–5.02; $p = 0.28$) for pedunculated vs. flat adenomas adjusted for size, villous component, and location, and corrected for correlation of risk within an individual patient. Patients with flat adenomas at initial colonoscopy were not at greater risk for advanced adenomas at surveillance compared with those with polypoid adenomas only, the odds ratio was 0.76 (95% CI 0.4–1.42; $p = 0.39$), adjusted for multiplicity, age, and family history of colorectal cancer. Flat adenomas identified in the National Polyp Study cohort at baseline were therefore not associated with a higher risk for high-grade dysplasia initially, or for advanced adenomas at surveillance.

Faecal occult blood testing during surveillance of patients after polypectomy[14]

Faecal occult blood test (FOBT) screening in the general population has been shown to reduce the mortality and incidence of colorectal cancer by detecting early-stage cancer and adenomas. It is often used clinically in patients who have had polypectomy and are in a colonoscopy surveillance programme. Considering the effectiveness of colonoscopy in detecting the majority of advanced neoplasia, we would expect FOBT to be of limited value in this setting. This study investigated the value of FOBT in patients having post-polypectomy surveillance colonoscopy. This study was conducted in the framework of the National Polyp Study. The efficacy of FOBT for detection of advanced adenomas was determined based on the FOBT results and the colonoscopy findings at the first surveillance colonoscopy. Of 973 newly diagnosed adenoma patients who had surveillance colonoscopy, 685 (70%) had an FOBT performed prior to their first surveillance colonoscopy. Average age was 62 years and 71% were men. An advanced adenoma was detected for 75 (11%) at the first surveillance colonoscopy and FOBT was positive for 69 (10%) of the patients. The sensitivity of FOBT for advanced adenomas was 21% (16 of 75); specificity was 91% (557 of 610), the positive predictive value was

23% (16 of 69), and negative predictive value 90% 557 of 616). As compared with patients with a negative test, those with a positive test had a significant risk of an advanced adenoma (odds ratio = 2.9 with 95% CI 1.5–5.3). Although a positive FOBT does indicate an increased risk for an advanced adenoma at surveillance, using this test in surveillance would detect few advanced adenomas (21%) and have many (77%) false-positive surveillance colonoscopies.

Association of hyperplastic polyps and advanced adenomas[15]

The major objective of the NPS was to determine the most effective surveillance of post-polypectomy patients for the control of large bowel cancer. Within the framework of this prospective, multicentre, randomized trial many questions can be addressed related to the management and natural history of polyps. One such question addressed is the possible association of hyperplastic polyps (HP) and adenomas (ADN). Classification of polyps included: ADN, HP, other (inflammatory, normal mucosa, miscellaneous). All ADN were graded for degree of dysplasia and presence of carcinoma. The number of patients screened was 5098, of whom 2047 had either ADN only (1690, 82%), HP only (178, 9%), or HP and ADN (179, 9%). The relative risk of having ADN with HP was 1.8 ($p < 0.001$). However, HP on the left (L) did not predict ADN on the right (proximal to the splenic flexure; relative risk of 1.2, n.s.). In patients with both HP and ADN the HP did not influence the anatomical distribution, histology, size, or mean number of ADN. Patients with ADN only had a mean of 1.8 ADN and patients with ADN and HP had a mean of 1.9 ADN and 1.6 HP. Patients with HP only had a mean number of 1.6. Although there is a small but significant association between HP and ADN in patients undergoing initial colonoscopy, L-sided HP do not predict R-sided ADN and the presence of HP does not influence the characteristics of ADN.

Dynamics of the adenoma–carcinoma sequence: MISCAN modelling of NPS data[16]

The National Polyp Study was a large longitudinal study that provides prospective data on the adenoma–carcinoma sequence. We examined the concordance between the observed data in the National Polyp Study and assumptions on the adenoma–carcinoma sequence using the MISCAN model in order to provide more insight into the natural history of colorectal cancer. The observed adenoma and cancer incidence in the National Polyp Study were compared with the simulated outcomes of the MISCAN-Colon model for the United States population based on expert opinion. Variants of this model were explored to identify assumptions that are consistent with the study observations. The high observed adenoma detection rates at surveillance and low observed versus expected colorectal cancer incidence in the National Polyp Study are best explained by assuming that high incidence rates of adenomas are accompanied by regression of adenomas. Applying the MISCAN model to the National Polyp Study data suggests that adenoma prevalence results from a dynamic process of both formation as well as regression of adenomas. Studies of primary prevention, screening and surveillance should consider these dynamics.

DISCUSSION

When the National Polyp Study was organized common clinical practice in the 1970s was to perform follow-up colonoscopy surveillance annually after colonoscopic polypectomy. The NPS demonstrated that clinicians could defer the first colonoscopy after polypectomy to 3 years in more than 90% of patients providing that the baseline colonoscopy cleared the colon of polyps with a high degree of confidence in an adequately prepared colon[8]. A small percentage of patients, those with malignant polyps, or where piecemeal or incomplete removal was done, of course needed follow-up at a shorter individualized time frame. These data provided the basis for guidelines published by the American Cancer Society and a US GI Consortium that recommended that follow-up surveillance colonoscopy be performed at 3-year intervals and not annually[17]. If this were followed nationally there would be a large savings in resources that could be shifted to the diagnostic work-up of patients with a positive FOBT or sigmoidoscopy. Subsequent observations by the NPS indicated that there are predictors that can be identified that could select patients at baseline for less intense or more intense surveillance, and that approximately 70% of post-polypectomy patients can have their subsequent follow-up at 5-year intervals, while reserving the 3-year intervals for those at increased risk of advanced adenomas[12]. These data, as well as data from other studies[19], provided the basis for risk stratification of patients at the time of polypectomy into lower and high risk groups for 3- or 5-year follow-up. This was incorporated initially into the GI Consortium updated guidelines (now the US Multisociety Colorectal Task Force)[18] and are more specifically and in a much more detailed manner being incorporated into combined American Cancer Society/US Multisociety Task Force guidelines that will soon be published[19].

Prior to the NPS studies it was widely believed that colorectal cancer arises from pre-existing adenomas[1], but it was never shown that removal of adenomas would result in a decreased incidence of colorectal cancer. This was demonstrated by the NPS[9] and led to the concept of screening colonoscopy which could screen, diagnose, treat with a single test and result in a reduced incidence of colorectal cancer. Although there are no randomized trials of screening colonoscopy with incidence or mortality as endpoints, there is sufficient evidence that this would result, based on early outcome findings of screening colonoscopy trials[20–22].

The NPS also demonstrated that the only effective follow-up surveillance after polypectomy is colonoscopy. The blinded comparison showed the double-contrast barium enema performed by expert radiology investigators to be very insensitive compared to colonoscopy, missing about 50% of large >1 cm adenomas[10]. We now know that colonoscopy also has a miss rate for adenomas and even for cancer[23–26]. It is critical for colonoscopy to be clearing the colon with high confidence, adequate preparation, and slow withdrawal in order to reduce this miss rate[27]. Additional observations in the NPS showed that FOBT in patients under colonoscopic surveillance were ineffective and resulted in additional unnecessary colonoscopies. An immunochemical FOBT fared no better[28]. The observation is being incorporated into present guidelines in which FOBT is discouraged in these patients.

It was of interest that, when the NPS review pathologist reviewed all adenomas using published pathological critical for flat adenomas, about one-third of all adenomas could be reclassified as flat[13]. They were originally called sessile by NPS endoscopists and pathologists. The NPS was able to demonstrate a 90% reduction in expected incidence of colorectal cancer without any special attention to flat adenomas and without the use of chromoendoscopy[9]. Only a small portion of flat adenomas are depressed and have advanced pathology. The importance of the flat adenomas is still controversial and requires further study[29].

Many other aspects of the NPS are described above in the results section, but the major impact of the NPS can be summarized as follows: (1) It has led to an evidence-based guidelines approach to surveillance of post-polypectomy patients, which is still evolving; (2) following these guidelines would help shift resources from surveillance to screening and diagnosis; (3) the demonstration that polypectomy prevents colon cancer has been a major driving force in the developing concept of screening colonoscopy; (4) the blinded methodology developed by NPS for the comparison of colonoscopy and DCBE has been used as a model for comparing optical colonoscopy and CT colonography[30], and the surveillance model of the NPS with the advanced adenoma endpoint has been adopted for studying the effects of fibre and chemoprevention on colonic adenomas[31]; (5) finally, the NPS data have provided the basis for a better understanding of the adenoma–carcinoma relationship, demonstrating that this is dynamic, with regression as well as progression of adenomas[16]. Further studies of the NPS data and further follow-up of this cohort will yield additional insights into the natural history of the adenomas–carcinoma relationship and the prevention colorectal cancer.

Acknowledgements

This work was supported by a grant (CA 26852) from the National Institutes of Health and sponsored by the American Gastroenterological Association, the American Society for Gastrointestinal Endoscopy, and the American College of Gastroenterology.

References

1. Winawer SJ. A quarter century of colorectal cancer screening: progress and prospects. J Clin Oncol. 2001;19:6s–12s.
2. Winawer SJ, Zauber AG, O'Brien MJ et al. The National Polyp Study: design, methods, and characteristics of patients with newly diagnosed patients. Cancer. 1992;70:1236–45.
3. O'Brien MJ, Winawer SJ, Zauber AG et al., National Polyp Study Workgroup. The National Polyp Study: Patient and polypcharacteristics associated with high-grade dysplasia in colorectal adenomas. Gastroenterology. 1990;98:371–9.
4. Hosmer DW Jr, Lemeshow S. Applied Logistic Regression. New York: John Wiley, 1989.
5. Armitage P, Berry G. Statistical Methods in Medical Research, 2nd edn. Oxford: Blackwell Scientific, 1987:411–17.
6. SAS/STAT User's Guide, version 6, 4th edn. Vols. 1, 2. Gary, NC: SAS Institute, 1989.
7. LR stepwise Logistic Regression: BMDP Statistical Software Manual, Vol. 2. Los Angeles: University of California Press, 1990:1013–46.
8. Winawer SJ, Zauber AG, O'Brien MJ et al. Randomizedcomparison of surveillance intervals after colonoscopic removal of newlydiagnosed adenomatous polyps. N Engl J Med. 1993;328:901–6.

9. Winawer SJ, Zauber AG, Ho MN, O'Brien MJ, Gottlieb LS. Prevention ofcolorectal cancer by colonoscopic polypectomy. N Engl J Med. 1993;329:1977–81.
10. Winawer SJ, Stewart ET, Zauber AG et al. A comparison ofcolonoscopy and double-contrast barium enema for surveillance afterpolypectomy. N Engl J Med. 2000;342:1766–72.
11. Winawer SJ, Zauber AG, Gerdes H et al. Risk ofcolorectal cancer in the families of patients with adenomatous polyps. N Engl J Med. 1996;334:82–7.
12. Zauber AG, Winawer SJ, Bond JH, Way JD, Schapiro M, et al. Can surveillanceintervals be lengthened following colonoscopic polypectomy? Gastroenterology. 1997;112:A50.
13. O'Brien MJ, Winawer SJ, Zauber AG, Bushey MT, Stemberg SS. Flat adenomasin the National Polyp Study: is there increased risk for high-grade dysplasiainitially or during surveillance. Clin Gastroenterol Hepatol. 2004;2:905–11.
14. Zauber AG, Winawer SJ, Bond JH et al.FOBT is of limited value in post-polypectomy colonoscopy surveillance. Gastroenterology. 2002:A-486,T1589.
15. Zauber A, Winawer SJ, Diaz B et. Al. The National Polyp Study (NPS): the association of colonic hyperplastic polyps andadenomas. Am J Gastroenterol. 1988;9:1060.
16. Loeve F, Boer R, Zauber AG et al. National Polyp Study Data: evidence of regression ofadenomas. Int J Cancer. 2004;111:633–9.
17. Winawer SJ, Fletcher RH, Miller L et al.Colorectal cancer screening: clinical guidelines and rationale. Gastroenterology. 1997;12:594–642.
18. Winawer SJ, Fletcher R, Rex D et al. Colorectal cancerscreening and surveillance: clinical guidelines and rationale – update based on new evidence. Gastroenterology. 2003;124:544–60.
19. Winawer S, Zauber A, Fletcher R. Post-polypectomy surveillance: a consensus Update by the US Multi-SocietyTask Force on Colorectal Cancer and the American Cancer Society. Gastroenterology. 2006 (In press).
20. Lieberman DA, Weiss DG, Bond JH et al. Use of colonoscopy toscreen asymptomatic adults for colorectal cancer. Veterans Affairs Cooperative Study Group 380. N Engl J Med. 2000;343:162–8.
21. Imperiale TF, Wagner DR, Lin CY et al. Risk of advanced proximalneoplasms in asymptomatic adults according to the distal colorectal findings. N Engl J Med. 2000:343:169–74.
22. Winawer SJ, Zauber AG, Church T et al. National Colonoscopy (NCS) Preliminary Results: a randomized controlled trial of general population screening colonoscopy. Gastroenterology. 2002;22A-480.
23. Hixson LJ, Fennerty MD, Sampliner RE, Garewal HS. Prospective blinded trialof the colonoscopic miss-rate of large colorectal polyps. Gastrointest Endosc. 1991;37:125–7.
24. Rex DK, Cutler CS, Lemmel GT et al. Colonoscopic miss rates of adenomas determined by back-to-backcolonoscopies. Gastroenterology. 1997;112:24–8.
25. Rex DK, Bond JH, Feld AD. Medical-legal risks of incidence cancers afterclearing colonoscopy. Am J Gastroenterol, 2001;96:952–7.
26. Dressier B, Paszat LF, Vinden C, Li C, He J, Rabeneck L. Colonoscopic missrates for right-sided colon cancer: a population-based analysis. Gastroenterology. 2004;127:452–6.
27. Rex DK, Bond JH, Winawer SJ et al. Quality inthe technical performance of colonoscopy and the continuous quality improvement process for colonoscopy: recommendations of the US Multisociety Task Force on Colorectal Cancer. Am J Gastroenterol. 2002;97:1296–308.
28. Bampton PA, Sandford JJ, Cole SR et al. Interval feacal occult blood testing in a colonoscopy based screening programmedetects additional pathology. Gut. 2005;54:803–6.
29. Kudo S, Tamara S, Nakajimo TT et al. Depressed type of colorectal cancer. Endoscopy. 1995;27:54–7.
30. Pickhardt PJ, Choi JR, Hwang I et al. Computedtomographic virtual colonoscopy to screen for colorectal neoplasia in asymptomatic adults. N Engl J Med. 2003;349:2191–200.
31. Robertson DJ, Greenberg ER, Beach M et al. Colorectal cancer in patients under close colonoscopic surveillance. Gastroenterology. 2005;129:34–41.

10
Colorectal cancer screening: cost-effectiveness and adverse events

D. LIEBERMAN

INTRODUCTION

Colorectal cancer (CRC) is the second leading cause of cancer death in North America. In 2005 there were 147 000 new cases, and 57 000 deaths in the United States[1]. Average-risk individuals have a 5–6% lifetime risk of developing CRC and a 2.5% risk of mortality. There is evidence that population screening can reduce both mortality and incidence of CRC.

To be effective screening must target appropriate populations, result in detection of important pathology at a curable stage, be accepted by patients, and be done with high quality. CRC screening presents an opportunity for early cancer detection and for cancer prevention. Most colorectal cancers evolve from pre-existing adenomas. This evolution from adenoma to cancer provides a unique opportunity for prevention if patients with pre-malignant neoplasia can be detected, and these lesions removed. There is compelling evidence that detection and removal of adenomas can prevent incident cancers[2,3]. Therefore, an important goal of CRC screening should be cancer prevention.

Despite compelling evidence of the effectiveness of screening, only 30–40% of individuals in the United States over 50 years old receive any of the recommended screening tests[4]. Among those who do receive screening, the quality of the screening programmes is quite variable. Ultimately, the effectiveness of screening depends on (1) patient compliance and (2) the quality of the screening programme. This chapter will review the current screening recommendations for average-risk individuals, and discuss adverse events and costs associated with each of the screening programmes.

RISK STRATIFICATION

Approximately 70% of patients who develop CRC are considered 'average risk', with a 5–6% lifetime risk of developing CRC, and a lifetime risk of death of 2.5%. Therefore, average risk is not low risk. It is important for primary-care providers to recognize patients with higher than average risk. Table 1 reviews

Table 1   Colorectal cancer risk stratification

Risk level	Percentage of all CRC	Recommendations for screening
High risk		
Familial polyposis	1	Sigmoidoscopy in teenage years
		Genetic screening can be considered
		Total colectomy if detected
		Surveillance for upper gastrointestinal malignancies
Hereditary non-polyposis colorectal cancer (HNPCC)	3–5	Colonoscopy in 3rd/4th decade at 2 year intervals
		Genetic screening can be considered
		Monitor for gynaecological malignancies
Chronic ulcerative colitis/Crohns colitis	<1	Colonoscopy every 2 years beginning at 8–10 years after onset of colitis
Moderate risk		
Familial risk: first-degree relative	15–20	Colonoscopy preferred
		Begin screening at an age 10 years younger than age of index case
Personal history of breast, uterine, ovarian cancer	<1	No specific recommendation
Average risk		
Age > 50 years	70–75	Begin screening at age 50

various high-risk conditions. Primary-care providers should ask two simple questions: (1) do you have a first-degree relative with CRC and (2) did that relative have CRC before age 50 years. If the answer to the second question is affirmative there should be suspicion of possible inherited germline mutation – either familial adenomatous polyposis (FAP) or hereditary non-polyposis colorectal cancer (HNPCC) syndrome. Recommendations for high-risk screening are outlined in Table 1 and are reviewed elsewhere[5].

AVERAGE-RISK SCREENING

An ideal screening test would be safe and non-invasive and would identify those patients most likely to develop CRC. None of the current recommended tests[5–8] meets this ideal standard; all have some advantages and limitations which will be discussed.

GUIAIC-BASED FAECAL OCCULT BLOOD TEST (gFOBT)

The evidence supporting the efficacy of gFOBT comes from large randomized controlled trials in asymptomatic populations[9–13]. These studies demonstrated that screened populations had CRC detected at an earlier and more curable stage than unscreened controls and, over time, this resulted in reduced mortality from CRC. The clinical trials achieved mortality reduction of 15–33%. If only adherent subjects are analysed the mortality reduction was 30–40%[9–11]. One of the studies further demonstrated a reduction in incidence which was attributed to adenoma detection and removal during the screening programme[3]. There are several important lessons from these studies:

Sensitivity

The gFOBT has been evaluated as a one-time test in two large screening colonoscopy studies in which asymptomatic patients received colonoscopy[14,15]. The rehydrated test detected 50% of invasive cancers, and 21% of advanced neoplasia[14]. The non-rehydrated test was positive in 13% of patients with cancer and 10% of patients with advanced neoplasia[15]. These studies highlight the importance of programmatic testing because of the poor detection rate with one-time testing. In the Minnesota study the programmatic test sensitivity for cancer was 92% for rehydrated and 81% for non-rehydrated FOBT[9]. Not all patients had colonoscopy, so the detection rate for advanced neoplasia is unknown.

Method of testing affects sensitivity and specificity

In the United States and Europe, most tests are performed using three stool samples (collected on three consecutive days) without rehydration. Prior studies have found that collection of three samples improves the likelihood of detecting important colon neoplasia compared to one sample. However, the three-sample collection creates a potential obstacle to adherence. In addition, gFOBT is not specific for human blood and will be positive if there is blood from consumed meat or if there is any bleeding from the upper gastrointestinal tract. These 'false-positive' tests result in potentially unnecessary colonoscopies. False-negative tests can occur with vitamin C. Therefore, many experts recommend that patients avoid red meat, peroxidase-containing foods and non-steroidal anti-inflammatory drugs prior to testing – creating yet another obstacle to adherence.

The rate of positive tests in asymptomatic populations is 2–6% for non-rehydrated gFOBT. The addition of water during the interpretation of the test (hydration) increases the positivity rate to as high as 15%[16]. The rehydrated test has a higher rate of sensitivity for CRC compared to non-rehydrated gFOBT, but at the cost of specificity[16]. Higher positivity rates result in higher rates of colonoscopy, with higher programmatic cost. Hemoccult SENSA is a more sensitive gFOBT which, like rehydrated Hemoccult, is associated with high positivity rates (5–13.5%)[16].

Recent data suggest that many physicians rely on a single in-office digital gFOBT instead of the 3-day at-home sample. The rationale for this approach is opportunistic, and reflects the poor rate of compliance with at-home testing. Many providers believe that the in-office test is better than no test at all ('better than nothing'). In the National Health Interview Survey, 32.5% of primary-care providers reported that they use in-office digital FOBT exclusively[17,18]. The VA Cooperative Study no. 380 determined the sensitivity of one-time

Table 2 Elements of FOBT screening programme

Proper performance of test: 3-day home sample
Adherence to initial test
Annual repeat testing after negative test
Follow-up of positive test – colonoscopy preferred
Colonoscopic surveillance after detection and removal of neoplasia
Cancer care for detected cancers or cancers which are discovered due to symptoms

digital gFOBT for detection of advanced neoplasia[19]. Less than 5% of patients with advanced neoplasia had a positive test. Moreover, a false-negative test may provide reassurance provided to patients, who may then decline to have a recommended form of screening. Therefore, the in-office digital gFOBT may be 'worse than nothing' because of low sensitivity and the impact of false reassurance on subsequent patient adherence to recommended testing.

Programmatic testing

The success of FOBT depends on implementation of a 'programme' (Table 2). In the clinical trials the tests were repeated either annually or biennially. One-time FOBT is relatively ineffective[14,15]. A successful FOBT programme must ensure that patients return for repeat testing annually. In clinical practice this is a significant challenge, even in the context of clinical trials. Adherence with repeat testing in patients who have the initial test drops to 50–75% in round two, and even lower in subsequent rounds. Therefore, practices which use FOBT should design reminder methods to ensure compliance with annual testing. Patients who do not adhere to a repeat testing programme should be strongly encouraged to have endoscopic screening.

Evaluation of positive gFOBT

There is clear evidence that patients with a positive gFOBT have a 3–4-fold increased likelihood of having either CRC or advanced neoplasia compared to patients with a negative test. All expert panels recommend that patients with a positive test have a complete structural examination of the colon – preferably with colonoscopy[5–8]. However, recent data from the National Health Interview Survey suggest that many health-care providers do not follow these recommendations[17]. A total of 1147 primary-care providers were asked what they recommend after a positive gFOBT; 30% of respondents recommended repeating the gFOBT. Among 925 physicians who did recommend follow-up testing, 22.5% recommended sigmoidoscopy alone. These data are alarming because they undermine the rationale for using gFOBT to identify higher-risk individuals who need colonoscopy.

Immunochemical FOBT (iFOBT)

There have been many efforts to improve the operating characteristics of a stool-based occult blood test. iFOBT uses antibodies specific for human globin in stool. There is no need for dietary or drug restrictions, which may help improve adherence with testing[20,21]. Test positivity rates of 3–5.9% are acceptable for population-based screening[16]. Test sensitivity for cancer ranges from 60% to 85%. A recent large study from Japan reported one-time iFOBT results in 21 805 patients with complete colonoscopy[22]. The test positivity rate was 5.6%; 79 patients (0.4%) had invasive cancer. The iFOBT was positive in 66% of cancer patients and in 20% of patients with adenomas >1 cm. The positive and negative predictive values were quite acceptable: 16% of patients with positive iFOBT had advanced neoplasia and 2.6% of patients with negative iFOBT had advanced neoplasia. A previous large study[23] found that iFOBT was more sensitive than gFOBT in a head-to-head comparison, while some other studies have been less impressive.

Adverse events

Programmatic effectiveness ultimately depends on compliance at every level of the screening programme (Table 2). To understand the impact of compliance we should consider likely mortality reduction based on realistic expectations of adherence. The randomized trials reported that CRC mortality reduction of up to 40% can be achieved in adherent patients. In clinical practice, adherence with initial testing rarely exceeds 75%, so that potential mortality reduction might be 30%. If 25% of patients who have initial testing do not have follow-up gFOBT after negative tests, mortality reduction could drop to 23%. If 25% of patients with positive tests do not have colonoscopy, the potential benefit of gFOBT would be further reduced to less than 20%.

Therefore, one of the most important adverse events with gFOBT is the false reassurance provided by a negative test. Patients and physicians need to understand that, if this programme is used for screening, it will be only effective if there are high levels of adherence with programmatic testing, and that any patient with a positive test should have colonoscopy.

FLEXIBLE SIGMOIDOSCOPY (FS)

Background

Evidence for the effectiveness of sigmoidoscopy comes from case–control studies[24,25] which found a 60% reduction in CRC mortality for cancers within reach of the sigmoidoscope in patients exposed to sigmoidoscopy. The studies did not demonstrate a benefit for patients with proximal cancers. However, if patients who have index adenomas of any size undergo colonoscopy, there is evidence that up to 70% of those with advanced neoplasia would be identified, including some patients with proximal advanced neoplasia[26,27]. The current recommendations call for repeat testing at 5 years[5–8], in contrast to a 10-year interval for screening colonoscopy (see section on colonoscopy below). Evidence supporting the interval is weak, and derived from a case–control study which found the risk of CRC was reduced over a 10-year period after screening sigmoidoscopy[24]. Studies have found low rates of advanced neoplasia or cancer within 5 years of a negative screening examination[28,29]. However, data from the PLCO study[30] have raised some questions about the interval. In this large study 0.8% of patients with a negative baseline test had advanced adenomas or cancer detected on a follow-up test within 3 years.

Quality control issues

A recent review of quality issues highlighted several important domains, including training, bowel preparation, technique, lesion recognition, complications, reporting and equipment processing[31]. I will focus on a few selected issues.

Definition of positive test.

What findings at sigmoidoscopy should result in referral for colonoscopy? There has been controversy over the past 15 years about the importance of small adenomas <10 mm seen in the distal colon. The debate has centred around whether such patients have an increased risk of proximal advanced neoplasia. Two recent studies used screening colonoscopy in asymptomatic subjects to estimate the outcome of performing sigmoidoscopy[26,27]. These studies, with more than 5000 patients, concluded that the finding of an adenoma of any size in the distal colon was associated with an increased risk of proximal advanced neoplasia, compared to patients who did not have polyps in the distal colon. However, some experts maintain that the absolute risk of advanced neoplasia is low, and may not justify the cost and risk of colonoscopy. The multi-society expert panel recommends that colonoscopy be considered if any adenoma is found in the distal colon at sigmoidoscopy, but suggests that this is an 'individual clinical decision'[5].

There has been considerable controversy about the significance of hyperplastic polyps in the distal colon. Current evidence suggests that these lesions are non-malignant, and are not harbingers of serious proximal pathology. The two large screening colonoscopy studies found that the risk of advanced proximal neoplasia (defined as adenoma ≥10 mm, adenoma with villous histology or high-grade dysplasia, or invasive cancer) in patients with distal hyperplastic polyps was similar to patients who had no polyps in the distal colon. These studies concluded that if the only finding in the distal colon was hyperplastic polyp(s), complete colonoscopy is not recommended. These recommendations have been endorsed by the multi-society panel[5].

Therefore, a key clinical decision may depend on the determination of histology of small distal polyps: if hyperplastic, no further evaluation is needed; if adenomatous, colonoscopy is recommended. Endoscopically, there are no reliable criteria that can discriminate a hyperplastic polyp (HP) from an adenomatous polyp (AP). Several studies have found that high-resolution chromoendoscopy with contrast agents and magnification can distinguish HP and AP with excellent sensitivity and specificity. Despite the success of these early studies, few endoscopists incorporate chromoendoscopy into their practice because of the additional time required to stain, and then examine, the colon segment. Even with sensitivity of more than 80%, these methods are not a perfect replacement for biopsy and histological evaluation. Therefore, another quality control issue for sigmoidoscopy rests on the decision to obtain a biopsy of small polyps to determine histology. Since the decision to proceed with colonoscopy depends on histology, small polyps encountered at sigmoidoscopy should be biopsied.

Adverse events

Adverse events associated with the performance of sigmoidoscopy are rare. Some patients with proximal malignancies will not be identified with sigmoidoscopy alone. There is some evidence that the prevalence of proximal neoplasms increases with advancing age. Therefore, sigmoidoscopy may be a less satisfactory screening test in elderly populations. A recent study found that sigmoidoscopy may be less effective in women than in men[39]. A large population-based study in the UK is still in progress and will address efficacy and safety of sigmoidoscopy[32].

IMAGING STUDIES

Background

Barium enema is included among the currently recommended screening tests for CRC. There are no effectiveness data in screening populations. The National Polyp Study[33] found that barium studies identified less than 50% of patients with polyps or lesions >10 mm. Recent studies have evaluated the accuracy of CT colonography (CTC) in screening populations, and this test has largely displaced barium studies as a potential screening test. Magnetic resonance imaging (MRI) is being evaluated in Europe, but few large studies have been performed. This discussion will highlight current CTC data and issues surrounding its use for screening.

Sensitivity

Three recent large studies have compared CTC with optical colonoscopy. Sensitivity, defined as detection of a patient with a polyp >10 mm, was 55%[34], 59%[35] and 94%[36], in the three studies. Earlier studies documented significant inter-observer variability[37], further emphasizing the importance of training. This variability has been attributed to training, computer software, labelling of stool and primary method of interpretation (2D vs 3D). These studies reflect the current state of the art. It is likely that very high sensitivity can be achieved with further improvements in methodology and training.

CTC issues

Threshold for positive test

Pickhardt et al.[36] found that up to 50% of asymptomatic patients had at least one polyp that can be detected with CTC. Many of these polyps will be hyperplastic or non-neoplastic. The threshold for referral to colonoscopy will be the key determinant of the overall cost of a CTC programme. If patients with small polyps are not referred, they may need to have follow-up CTC to monitor growth of polyps. Programmatic costs from referral to colonoscopy or repeat CTC will need to be considered in any cost analysis.

Bowel preparation

Currently, a complete bowel prep is required for CTC, to reduce the likelihood of false-positive examinations. In the future it may be possible to have a prep-less examination by labelling stool and subtracting stool from the analysis. The requirement of a bowel prep raises issues with patient compliance. If patients have a positive test, and are referred for colonoscopy, they will require a second bowel prep (unless the procedure can be performed immediately after CTC). Patients, once informed of the possible need for two bowel preps, may not prefer CTC.

Radiation

The actual radiation dosing for CTC is low, and in the future may be reduced further. However, concern has been raised that if asymptomatic patients have repeat CTC every few years, the cumulative dose of radiation could reach levels associated with increased cancer risk. A recent review of this subject suggests that the radiation risk is low, but the risk of radiation-induced cancer may be roughly equivalent to the risk of perforation of the colon during colonoscopy[38].

Extracolonic findings

When abdominal CT is performed in asymptomatic subjects, extracolonic findings are common[36]. Although most of these incidental findings are clinically unimportant, they can lead to further tests, which can be costly and associated with morbidity. In rare cases important new asymptomatic lesions (such as renal cell carcinoma) may be discovered. Cost analyses of CTC should include the cost of evaluation of extracolonic lesions.

Summary of imaging

CTC offers a new modality for colon imaging that will probably be very accurate as technology and training improve. However, the test will not be cost-effective unless physicians and patients are comfortable with ignoring diminutive polyps <6 mm. For patients with polyps of 6–9 mm a choice of repeat CTC or colonoscopy will need to be considered. Further study is needed to determine the appropriate interval for repeat CTC if colonoscopy is not performed. Patients with polyps > 9 mm will probably be referred for colonoscopy.

STOOL DNA TESTS

Several important genetic mutations have been associated with colon carcinogenesis. Since colonic cells die and are replaced, some of this mutated DNA is excreted in stool. Recent studies have utilized polymerase chain reaction (PCR) methodology to identify a panel of mutations associated with CRC in stool samples – searching for a genetic 'needle in the haystack'. These proof-of-principle studies demonstrate that mutations, when present, can be detected in stool. The largest study found that stool DNA was positive in 52% of cancers, but only 18% of patients with advanced neoplasia[15]. Further study is needed to improve the detection rate of the test.

COLONOSCOPY

Evidence of effectiveness

Ideally, colonoscopy would be reserved for those patients who have a less-invasive screening test that is positive. However, as noted above, each of the current screening tests has significant limitations in detection of patients with advanced neoplasia. Large screening colonoscopy studies have been performed which have demonstrated feasibility of colonoscopy screening in average-risk, asymptomatic populations, when performed by fully trained endoscopists. These trials have highlighted some of the limitations of sigmoidoscopy[26,27,39] and gFOBT[14] noted above.

There are no long-term studies which have demonstrated the ability of primary colonoscopy screening to reduce mortality or incidence of CRC. All of the current evidence is indirect, albeit compelling. A case–control study[40] found reduced mortality associated with endoscopic screening. The gFOBT studies used colonoscopy to evaluate patients with positive screening tests. The subsequent mortality incidence reduction was attributed to colonoscopic detection of early cancers and removal of premalignant adenomas. The sigmoidoscopy studies found that CRC mortality was reduced in that portion of the colon which was examined. The implication is that, if more colons were examined, the benefit would be greater. Finally, the National Polyp Study (NPS) performed colonoscopy and polypectomy in 1418 subjects with adenomas; the subsequent incidence rate of CRC over the next 6 years was reduced by 76–90%, compared to three reference populations[2]. Although this does not prove that screening colonoscopy would reduce mortality by this level, the NPS does demonstrate that polypectomy can prevent cancer incidence.

Sensitivity

Colonoscopy is widely regarded as the most accurate test for detection of colon neoplasia. Most studies have used colonoscopy as the 'gold standard' against which other modalities are compared. The recent CTC studies have provided a new method for evaluating accuracy of colonoscopy[34–36]. In these studies the patients had CTC first, and then optical colonoscopy. After the optical evaluation of segments of the colon, the results of CTC were 'unblinded'. If a polyp was seen on CTC the segment was re-examined. If the polyp was detected on the second look, it was considered a missed lesion with optical colonoscopy. Using this method of segmental unblinding, the three large studies found that the miss-rate for polyps > 10 mm ranged from 2% to 12%. The miss-rate is further highlighted by the finding of early interval cancers after complete colonoscopy and polypectomy in several studies. Studies designed to evaluate chemoprevention with aspirin, calcium or diet performed a baseline clearing colonoscopy and then follow-up examinations within 3 years. The rate of cancers at 3 years in these trials was 0.7%, with a range of 1.7–2.4 per 1000 person-years of follow-up[41–43]. It is likely that some of the interval cancers were lesions that were not detected at the baseline examination. Therefore, although colonoscopy is the most accurate test for colon neoplasia, it is not perfect, even when performed by experienced endoscopists.

Safety

Colonoscopy is an invasive test with a risk of perforation and significant bleeding of approximately 3 per 1000 procedures. In addition, cardiopulmonary events may also occur. In the United States, conscious sedation, and sometimes deep sedation, are used, and sedation-related complications can occur. The actual risk of colonoscopy in community practice is largely unknown. Few studies have evaluated adverse events within 30 days of colonoscopy[44]. A community-based study of 30-day complications is currently in progress (Cynthia Ko, personal communication). In average-risk, asymptomatic patients, these risks must be balanced against the potential benefit of early cancer detection or cancer prevention.

Cost

Colonoscopy has a high 'up-front' cost, relative to other screening programmes. However, cost should be examined programmatically. For example, gFOBT has a low cost for initial screening. However, when analysed over a lifetime of annual screening, the programmatic costs are relatively similar to the costs of screening with colonoscopy every 10 years. The decision models show that colonoscopy, while more costly than other forms of screening (when calculated as cost per added year of quality life), is likely to be associated with higher rates of cancer prevention than any other programme.

Quality

The success of colonoscopy as a primary screening test, or a secondary test after an initial test, depends on quality. Quality indicators for colonoscopy have recently been reviewed by an expert panel[45].

CRC COST-EFFECTIVENESS

Most analyses of cost-effectiveness have used decision modelling methodology. A recent workshop by the Institute of Medicine reviewed several models[46]. When similar assumptions are applied, each of the screening programmes is cost-effective, relative to other medical interventions. FOBT programme costs are generally lower than others, but result in less cancer prevention than a more costly colonoscopy programme. The modellers assumed high rates of compliance in FOBT programmes, which may not be representative of what happens in clinical practice. Any reduction in adherence at any level of the FOBT programme (Table 2) would result in a less effective programme.

Most of the decision models have analysed programmes which utilize one screening test over a lifetime. The use of hybrid programmes in clinical practice is not known. For example, sigmoidoscopy or FOBT might be used in the sixth decade when absolute CRC risk is low, and then colonoscopy in the seventh decade as risk increases. Patients who do not comply with annual FOBT should be offered endoscopic screening. The efficacy of such programmes is unknown, but they are likely to be efficacious if patient adherence can be achieved.

SUMMARY

There is compelling evidence that CRC screening in average-risk populations is effective: screening can reduce CRC mortality and incidence. Moreover, the natural history of CRC provides a unique opportunity for cancer prevention, if patients with advanced adenomas can be identified, and those adenomas removed. Despite this evidence, less than 50% of individuals over age 50 years receive recommended screening in the United States. Primary-care providers play a key role in CRC screening. There is evidence that patients are much more likely to have screening if there is a recommendation from the primary provider. Each screening programme has advantages and limitations. The menu of screening options may seem to be confusing, and present a barrier to screening. However, patients and providers should understand that screening with any of the current tests is better than no screening. Providers should ensure that screening is performed with high quality to ensure the maximal effectiveness of the selected screening programme.

References

1. Jemal A, Murray T, Samuels A et al. Cancer statistics 2005. CA Cancer J Clin. 2005;55:10–30.
2. Winawer SJ, Zauber AG, Ho MN et al. Prevention of colorectal cancer by colonoscopic polypectomy. N Engl J Med. 1993;329:1977–81.
3. Mandel JS, Church TR, Bond JH et al. The effect of fecal occult-blood screening on the incidence of colorectal cancer. N Engl J Med. 2000;343:1603–7.
4. Centers for Disease Control and Prevention. Trends in screening for colorectal cancer – United States, 1997 and 1999. Morb Mortal Wkly Rep. 2001;50:162–6.
5. Winawer S, Fletcher R, Rex D et al. Colorectal cancer screening and surveillance: clinical guidelines and rationale – update based on new evidence. Gastroenterology. 2003;124:544–60.
6. Pignone M, Rich M, Teutsch SM, Berg AO, Lohr KN. Screening for colorectal cancer in adults at average risk: a summary of the evidence for the US Preventive Services Task Force. Ann Intern Med. 2002;137:132–41.
7. Smith RA, Cokkinides V, Eyre HJ. American Cancer Society guidelines for the early detection of cancer 2003. Cancer J Clin. 2003;53:27–43.
8. Rex DK, Johnson DA, Lieberman DA, Burt RW, Sonnenberg A. Colorectal cancer prevention 2000: screening recommendations of the American College of Gastroenterology. Am J Gastroenterol. 2000;95:868–77.
9. Mandel JS, Bond JH, Church TR et al. Reducing mortality from colorectal cancer by screening for fecal occult blood. N Engl J Med. 1993;328:1365–71.
10. Hardcastle JD, Chamberlain J, Robinson MHE et al. Randomized, controlled trial of fecal occult blood screening for colorectal cancer. Lancet. 1996;148:1472–7.
11. Kronborg, O, Fenger C, Olsen J, Jorgensen OD, Sondergaard O. Randomized study of screening for colorectal cancer with fecal occult blood test. Lancet. 1996;148:1467–71.
12. Jorgensen OD, Kronborg O, Fenger C. A randomised study of screening for colorectal cancer using faecal occult blood testing: results after 13 years and seven biennial screening rounds. Gut. 2002;50:29–32.
13. Faivre J, Dancourt V, Lejeune C et al. Reduction in colorectal cancer mortality by fecal occult blood screening in a French controlled study. Gastroenterology. 2004;126:1674–80.
14. Lieberman DA, Weiss DG and the VA Cooperative Study Group 380. One-time screening for colorectal cancer with combined fecal occult-blood testing and examination of the distal colon. N Engl J Med. 2001;345:555–60.
15. Imperiale TF, Ransohoff DE, Itzkowitz SH, Turnbull BA, Ross ME. Colorectal Cancer Study Group. Fecal DNA vs fecal occult blood for colorectal cancer screening in an average-risk population. N Engl J Med. 2004;351:2704–14.
16. Young GP, St John JB, Winawer SJ, Rozen P. Choice of fecal occult blood tests for colorectal cancer screening: recommendations based on performance characteristics in population studies. Am J Med. 2002;97:2499–507.
17. Nadel MR, Shapiro JA, Klabunde CN et al. A national survey of primary care physicians' methods for screening for fecal occult blood. Ann Intern Med. 2005;142:86–94.
18. Klabunde CN, Frame PS, Meadow A, Jones E, Nadel M, Vernon SW. A national survey of primary care physicians' colorectal cancer screening recommendations and practices. Prev Med. 2003;36:352–62.
19. Collins JF, Lieberman DA, Durbin TE, Weiss DG. Accuracy of screening for fecal occult blood on a single stool sample obtained by digital rectal examination: a comparison with recommended sampling practice. Ann Intern Med. 2005;142:81–5.
20. Cole SR, Young GP. Participation in fecal occult blood test-based screening for colorectal cancer is reduced by dietary restriction. Med J Aust. 2001;175:195–8.
21. Nakama H, Zhang B, Fattah ASMA. A cost-effective analysis of the optimum number of stool specimens collected for immunochemical occult blood screening for colorectal cancer. Eur J Cancer. 2000;36:647–50.
22. Morikawa T, Kato J, Yamaji Y, Wada Y, Mitsushima T, Shiratori Y. A comparison of the immunochemical fecal occult blood test and total colonoscopy in the asymptomatic population. Gastroenterology. 2005;129:422–8.
23. Allison JE, Tekawa IS, Ransom LJ, Adrian AL. A comparison of fecal-occult blood tests for colorectal cancer screening. N Engl J Med. 1996;336:155–9.

24. Selby JV, Friedman GD, Quesenberry CP Jr, Weiss NS. A case–control study of screening sigmoidoscopy and mortality from colorectal cancer. N Engl J Med. 1992;326:653–7.

25. Newcomb PA, Norfleet RG, Storer BE, Surawicz TS, Marcus PM. Screening sigmoidoscopy and colorectal cancer mortality. J Natl Cancer Inst. 1992;84:1572–5.

26. Lieberman DA, Weiss DG, Bond JH, Ahnen DJ, Garewal H, Chejfec G and VACSP Group no. 380. Use of colonoscopy to screen asymtomatic adults for colorectal cancer. N Engl J Med. 2000;343:162–8.

27. Imperiale TF, Wagner DR, Lin CY, Larkin GR, Rogge JD, Ransohoff DF. Risk of advanced proximal neoplasms in asymptomatic adults according to the distal colorectal findings. N Engl J Med. 2000;343:169–74.

28. Rex DK, Cummings OW, Helper DJ et al. 5-year incidence of adenomas after negative colonoscopy in asymptomatic average-risk persons. Gastroenterology. 1996;111:1178–81.

29. Doria-Rose VP, Levin TR, Selby JV, Newcomb PA, Richert-Boe KE, Weiss NS. The incidence of colorectal cancer following a negative screening sigmoidoscopy: implications for screening interval. Gastroenterology. 2004;127:714–22.

30. Schoen RE, Pinsky PF, Weissfeld JL et al for PLCO Group. Results of repeat sigmoidoscopy 3 years after a negative sigmoidoscopy. J Am Med Assoc. 2003;290:41–8.

31. Ashley OS, Nadel M, Ransohoff DF. Achieving quality in flexible sigmoidoscopy screening for colorectal cancer. Am J Med. 2001;111:643–53.

32. Atkin W, Rogers P, Cardwell C et al. Wide variation in adenoma detection rates at screening flexible sigmoidoscopy. Gastroenterology. 2004;126:1247–56.

33. Winawer SJ, Stewart ET, Zauber AG et al., NPS Workgroup. A comparison of colonoscopy and double-contrast barium enema for surveillance after polypectomy. N Engl J Med. 2000;342:1766–72.

34. Cotton PB, Durkalski VL, Pineau BC et al. Computed tomographic colonography (virtual colonoscopy): a multicenter comparison with standard colonoscopy for detection of colorectal neoplasms. J Am Med Assoc. 2004;291:1713–19.

35. Rockey DC, Paulson E, Niedzwiecki D et al. Analysis of air contrast barium enema, computed tomographic colonography and colonoscopy: prospective comparison. Lancet. 2005;365:305–11.

36. Pickhardt PJ, Choi R, Hwang I et al. Computed tomographic virtual colonoscopy to screen for colorectal neoplasia in asymptomatic adults. N Engl J Med. 2003;349:2191–200.

37. Johnson CD, Harmsen WS, Wilson LA et al. Prospective blinded evaluation of computerized tomographic colonography for screen detection of colorectal polyps. Gastroenterology. 2003;125:311–19.

38. Brenner DJ, Georgsson MA. Mass screening with CT colonography: should the radiation exposure be of concern? Gastroenterology. 2005;129:328–37.

39. Schoenfeld P, Cash B, Flood A et al. Colonoscopic screening of average-risk women for colorectal neoplasia. N Engl J Med. 2005;352:2061–8.

40. Muller AD, Sonnenberg A. Prevention of colorectal cancer by flexible endoscopy and polypectomy: a case–control study of 32 702 veterans. Ann Intern Med. 1995;123:904–10.

41. Schatzkin A, Lanza E, Corle D et al. and the Polyp Prevention Trial Study Group. Lack of effect of a low-fat, high-fiber diet on the recurrence of colorectal adenomas. N Engl J Med. 2000;342:1149 55.

42. Alberts DS, Martinez ME, Roe DJ et al. and the Phoenix Colon Cancer Prevention Physicians Network. Lack of effect of a high-fiber cereal supplement on the recurrence of colorectal adenomas. N Engl J Med. 2000;342:1156–62.

43. Robertson DJ, Greenberg ER, Beach M et al. Colorectal cancer in patients under close colonoscopic surveillance. Gastroenterology. 2005;129:34–41.

44. Nelson DB, McQuaid KR, Bond JH et al. Procedural success and complications of large-scale screening colonoscopy. Gastrointest Endosc. 2002;55:307–14.

45. Rex DK, Bond JH, Winawer S et al. Quality in the technical performance of colonoscopy and the continuous quality improvement process for colonoscopy: recommendations of the US Multi-Society task force on colorectal cancer. Am J Gastroenterol. 2002;97:1296–308.

46. Pignone M, Russell L, Wagner J, editors. Economic models of colorectal cancer screening in average-risk adults. Institute of Medicine Workshop. National Academic Press, 2005.

11
Detecting dysplasias in ulcerative colitis

R. KIESSLICH and M. F. NEURATH

INTRODUCTION

Long-standing ulcerative colitis (UC) is associated with an increased risk for the development of colon carcinoma and requires surveillance colonoscopy. In contrast to sporadic colorectal cancer, preneoplastic lesions in UC grow flat in the mucosa and thus represent a challenge to the endoscopist. In this chapter we will discuss recent developments in endoscopy for an enhanced detection rate of intraepithelial neoplasias in UC. In particular, recent data suggest that chromoendoscopy with methylene blue or indigo carmine is evolving as the new standard for surveillance colonoscopy in UC patients.

SCREENING PROCEDURES FOR UC

UC is an inflammatory bowel disease of unknown origin that causes chronic intestinal inflammation[1-7]. The disease is characterized by erosions and ulcer formation of the colon resulting in recurrent bleeding and diarrhoea[3]. Long-standing UC is associated with an increased risk for development of colitis-associated colon cancer[8-11]. Established risk factors for colitis-associated colon cancer in UC comprise the extent and severity of the disease as well as the presence of primary sclerosing cholangitis[12-14].

Based on the increased risk for colitis-associated colon carcinoma, surveillance colonoscopy in UC is important to detect early neoplastic lesions such as intraepithelial neoplasias[12,15]. However, many early lesions in UC grow flat in the mucosa and are easily overlooked by routine colonoscopy. Based on this finding 30–50 random biopsies have been recommended during surveillance colonoscopy. However, this approach is time consuming and bears the risk of overlooking relevant lesions.

CHROMOENDOSCOPY USING DYES

Recently, chromoendoscopy has been suggested as an alternative to colonoscopy with random biopsies for surveillance of UC patients[15,16]. During chromoendoscopy dye-spraying of the entire colorectal mucosa in UC helps to unmask mucosal irregularities, reducing the risk of overlooking subtle abnormalities. For chromoendoscopy, 100 ml of 0.47% indigo carmine or 100 ml of methylene blue 0.1% is prepared before the procedure, and drawn into 20 ml syringes. A dye-spray catheter is then inserted down the instrumentation channel of the colonoscope. An assistant subsequently squeezes the syringe, generating a fine mist of dye, which is then painted onto the mucosa by withdrawing the colonoscope in spiral fashion. Segments of 5–15 cm should be sprayed in clinical practice. Once a segment has been sprayed, excess dye is suctioned, and the colonoscope reinserted to the proximal extent of the segment. A stable staining pattern occurs after absorption of the dye. The glandular openings of the crypts appear as white spots surrounded by blue lines in a hexagonal fashion.

Several prospective studies have analysed the potential benefit for chromoendoscopy in UC. In a prospective, randomized study chromoendoscopy with 0.1% methylene blue was superior to detect intraepithelial neoplasias (IN) and colon cancer as compared to colonoscopy with random biopsies[17]. This finding was underlined by a study from Hurlstone and colleagues in which chromoendoscopy with indigo carmine resulted in increased detection of IN as compared to colonoscopy with random biopsies[18]. Similarly, Rutter et al.[19] and Matsumoto et al.[20] reported the successful use of chromoendoscopy for surveillance colonoscopy in UC. Taken together, these data indicate that chromoendoscopy in patients with long-standing UC might be a new evolving standard for surveillance colonoscopy[15]. Collectively, these data indicate that chromoendoscopy leads to a significant increase in the diagnostic yield of intraepithelial neoplasias in UC and is superior to standard colonoscopy with random biopsies.

Olliver and colleagues[21] recently raised some concerns about the intravital dye methylene blue. In patients with Barrett oesophagus they found oxidative DNA damage after chromoendoscopy (as measured by single-cell gel electrophoresis) and argued that methylene blue together with white light during endoscopy could also be a risk for patients to drive carcinogenesis. Therefore, the question arises whether methylene blue-aided chromoendoscopy may contribute to the carcinogenic process in UC, and leads to an increase of intraepithelial neoplasias in follow-up[21-25]. However, the design of the study by Olliver et al. must be substantially criticized due to the absence of a control group with light exposure only. Furthermore, the results from the distal oesophagus cannot be simply translated to the colon. In a follow-up study after chromoendoscopy with methylene blue in patients with UC, fewer lesions could be demonstrated upon previous chromoendoscopies as compared to patients who were screened by standard colonoscopy[22]. These data suggest that chromoendoscopy with methylene blue is a safe and highly effective approach for the detection of flat colonic lesions in UC. The reported increase of DNA lesions upon methylene blue–light treatment is unlikely to have

Table 1 Seven guidelines (SURFACE) for chromoendoscopy in UC

1.	Strict patient selection: patients with histologically proven UC and at least 8 years duration in clinical remission; avoid patients with active disease
2.	Unmask the mucosal surface: an excellent bowel preparation is needed. Remove mucus and remaining fluid in the colon when necessary
3.	Reduce peristaltic waves: when drawing back the endoscope a spasmolytic agent should be used (if necessary)
4.	Full-length staining of the colon: perform full-length staining of the colon (panchromoendoscopy) in UC rather than local staining
5.	Augmented detection with dyes: intravital staining with 0.1% indigo carmine or methylene blue should be used to unmask flat lesions more frequently than with conventional colonoscopy
6.	Crypt architecture analysis: all lesions should be analysed according to the pit-pattern lesions, staining patterns III–V suggest the presence of intraepithelial neoplasias and carcinomas
7.	Endoscopic targeted biopsies: perform targeted biopsies of all mucosal alterations, particularly of circumscript lesions with staining patterns indicative of intraepithelial neoplasias and carcinomas (pit-patterns III–V)

biological significance *in vivo*, and unwanted side-effects appear to be negligible in view of the advantages of the method.

SUMMARY AND OUTLOOK

Based on various prospective controlled studies, pan-colonic dye-spray during colonoscopic surveillance helps to detect flat areas of dysplasia or superficial cancer in the colon of patients with long-standing extensive UC. Thus, chromoendoscopy or alternative techniques such as narrow-band imaging with smart biopsies may replace random biopsies in the near future. However, chromoendoscopy should not be performed if the patient is allergic to the dye (e.g. methylene blue). Furthermore, surveillance colonoscopy may be inappropriate in patients with multiple post-inflammatory polyps throughout the colon. Finally, seven important points should be considered when doing chromoendocopy (see SURFACE guidelines, Table 1). Particular attention should be paid to strict patient selection, excellent bowel preparation, reduction of peristaltic waves, full-length staining of the colon, augmented detection with dyes, crypt architecture analysis and targeted biopsies.

References

1. Friedman S, Blumberg RS. Inflammatory bowel disease. In: Harrison's Principles of Internal Medicine, 15th edn. New York, London: Saunders, 1999:1679–91.
2. Strober W, Neurath MF. Immunological diseases of the gastrointestinal tract. In: Rich RR, editor. Clinical Immunology. St. Louis: Mosby, 1995:1401–28.
3. Karp LC, Targan SR. Ulcerative colitis. In: Ogra PL, editor. Mucosal Immunology, 2nd edn. New York: Academic Press, 1999:1047–53.

4.   Hanauer SB. Medical therapy for ulcerative colitis 2004. Gastroenterology. 2004;126:1582–92.
5.   Bouma G, Strober W. The immunological and genetic basis of inflammatory bowel disease. Nat Rev Immunol. 2003;3:521–33.
6.   Neurath MF, Finotto S, Glimcher LH. The role of Th1/Th2 polarization in mucosal immunity. Nature Med. 2002;8:567–73.
7.   Podolsky DK. Inflammatory bowel disease. N Engl J Med. 2002;347:417–29.
8.   Bernstein CN. The color of dysplasia in ulcerative colitis. Gastroenterology. 2003;124:1135–8.
9.   Heuschen HA, Hinz U, Allemeyer EH et al. Backwash ileitis is strongly associated with colorectal carcinoma in ulcerative colitis. Gastroenterology. 2001;120:841–7.
10. Butt JH, Konishi F, Morson BC, Lennard-Jones JE. Macroscopic lesions in dysplasia and carcinoma complicating ulcerative colitis. Dig Dis Sci. 1983;28:18–26.
11. Ekbom A, Helmick C, Zack M, Adami HO. Ulcerative colitis and colorectal cancer. N Engl J Med. 1990;323:1228–33.
12. Eaden JA, MayberryJF. Colorectal cancer complicating ulcerative colitis: a review. Am J Gastroenterol. 2000;95:2710–19.
13. Eaden JA, Abrams KR, Mayberry JF. The risk of colorectal cancer in ulcerative colitis: a meta-analysis. Gut. 2001;48:526–35.
14. Rutter M, Saunders B, Wilkinson K et al. Severity of inflammation is a risk factor for colorectal neoplasia in ulcerative colitis. Gastroenterology. 2004;126:451–9.
15. Kiesslich R, Neurath MF. Surveillance colonoscopy in ulcerative colitis: magnifying chromoendoscopy in the spotlight. Gut. 2004;53:165–67.
16. Kiesslich R, Jung M, DiSario JA, Galle PR, Neurath MF. Perspectives of chromo and magnifying endoscopy: how, how much, when, and whom should we stain? J Clin Gastroenterol. 2004;38:7–13.
17. Kiesslich R, Fritsch J, Holtmann M et al. 2003. Methylene blue-aided chromoendoscopy for the detection of intraepithelial neoplasia and colon cancer in ulcerative colitis. Gastroenterology. 2003;124:880–8.
18. Hurlstone DP, McAlindon ME, Sanders DS, Koegh R, Lobo AJ, Cross SS. Further validation of high-magnification chromoscopic-colonoscopy for the detection of intraepithelial neoplasia and colon cancer in ulcerative colitis. Gastroenterology. 2004;126:376–8.
19. Rutter MD, Saunders BP, Schofield G, Forbes A, Price AB, Talbot IC. Pancolonic indigo carmine dye spraying for the detection of dysplasia in ulcerative colitis. Gut. 2004;53:256–60.
20. Matsumoto T, Nakamura S, Jo Y, Yao T, Iida M. Chromoscopy might improve diagnostic accuracy in cancer surveillance for ulcerative colitis. Am J Gastroenterol. 2003;98:1827–33.
21. Olliver JR, Wild CP, Sahay P, Dexter S, Hardie LJ. Chromoendoscopy with methylene blue and associated DNA damage in Barrett's oesophagus. Lancet. 2003;362:373–4.
22. Kiesslich R, Burg J, Kaina B, Galle PR, Neurath MF. Safety and efficacy of methylene blue-aided chromoendoscopy in ulcerative colitis: a prospective pilot study upon previous chromoendoscopies, Abstract and oral presentation DDW 2004, New Orleans, USA.
23. Epe B, Hegler J, Wild D. Singlet oxygen as an ultimately reactive species in Salmonella typhimurium DNA damage induced by methylene blue/visible light. Carcinogenesis. 1989;10:2019–24.
24. Pflaum M, Kielbassa C, Garmyn B, Epe B. Oxidative DNA damage induced by visible light in mammalian cells: extent, inhibition by antioxidants and genotoxic effects. Mutation Res. 1998;408:137–46.
25. Friedberg EC, Walker GC, Siede W. DNA Repair and Mutagenesis. Washington, ASM Press, 1995:124–36.

Section V
Colorectal cancer: prevention

Chair: A. REINACHER-SCHICK and G. TRENN

12
A statistical model for post-polypectomy surveillance: a virtual alternative to virtual colonoscopy?

A. G. ZAUBER, I. VOGELAAR, M. VAN BALLEGOOIJEN, R. BOER, F. LOEVE, J. D. F. HABBEMA and S. J. WINAWER

INTRODUCTION

Although colorectal cancer is the second leading cause of cancer death in the United States[1], it can be prevented with screening[2-4]. The most frequent neoplasms found during colorectal screening are adenomatous polyps[4-7]. Removal of these lesions has been shown to reduce the risk of future colorectal cancer and advanced adenomas[8-15]. To further minimize the risk of colorectal cancer, patients with adenomas are usually placed into a surveillance programme of periodic colonoscopy to remove missed synchronous and new metachronous adenomas and cancers[16-19]. A large number of patients with adenomas are now being discovered as a result of the dramatic increase in screening colonoscopy, and this places a huge burden on medical resources applied to surveillance[20-22]. Therefore, there is a need for increased efficiency of surveillance colonoscopy practices in order to decrease the cost, risk, and over-utilization of resources for unnecessary examinations[23].

Most of the literature on surveillance for adenoma patients is from historical prospective analyses of registry data or from chemoprevention randomized controlled trials[8,10,15,24-37]. However, in the registry data there are generally variable follow-up periods and incomplete compliance. In the chemoprevention studies in adenoma patients there is standardized surveillance and high compliance, but the surveillance period is relatively short[23]. The National Polyp Study (NPS) was one of the few clinical trials to assess how adenoma patients should be managed for surveillance with follow-up more frequently (1 and 3 years following initial polypectomy) or less frequently (3 years following polypectomy) and demonstrated that a 3-year wait until first surveillance colonoscopy provided comparable protection as surveillance at 1-year and 3-year surveillance colonoscopy provided that the initial colonoscopy examination was of high quality[33]. The NPS also had surveillance follow-up to 6 years after the initial polypectomy. Consequently further examination of the NPS surveillance findings would be pertinent to assess more efficient uses of surveillance resources.

The NPS demonstrated that detection and removal of adenomatous polyps is associated with a 76–90% reduced risk of subsequent colorectal cancer[8]. This incidence reduction was achieved with initial polypectomy and surveillance colonoscopy for patients with adenomas in a randomized controlled trial comparing surveillance intervals of 1, 3 and 6 years versus at 3 and 6 years post-polypectomy. Of importance is deciding whether the incidence reduction was due to the initial or surveillance colonoscopies, or to both, and how long the interventions had an effect. We cannot directly observe the separate effects of the initial and surveillance colonoscopy because all adenoma patients received both initial and surveillance colonoscopy. However, we can use microsimulation modelling to assess the separate effects. We also can use microsimulation modelling to address the important question of whether all patients require 3-year surveillance or whether the surveillance colonoscopies could be lengthened for lower-risk patients. An additional issue is whether virtual colonoscopy could be used for the surveillance for lower-risk patients without diminishing the incidence reduction achieved.

In this chapter we demonstrate how we can use microsimulation modelling to assess effective and efficient surveillance strategies for adenoma patients. We describe the MISCAN microsimulation model for colorectal cancer and show how it can be used to extrapolate the NPS results to assess the effect of longer surveillance times for different risk groups.

METHODS

MISCAN microsimulation model for colorectal cancer

MISCAN-Colon is a microsimulation programme for the natural history of colorectal cancer and the effect of interventions along the adenoma–carcinoma sequence. MISCAN is an acronym of MIcroSimulation Screening ANalysis, and was developed for colorectal cancer by the Department of Public Health at Erasmus MC, the Netherlands, in cooperation with the National Cancer Institute (NCI) in the United States to evaluate population-based interventions to reduce colorectal cancer incidence and mortality. This work started in September 1995, resulting in the 1998 expert model[38–40]. Further developments in the model are currently under way as part of the Cancer Incidence and Surveillance Network (CISNET) sponsored by the US National Cancer Institute[41].

MISCAN-Colon consists of three parts: demography, natural history, and intervention effects. MISCAN-Colon first generates a series of individual life histories in the demography part to form a population according to the demography parameters (e.g. the birth and life table) by sex and race. Data on each person in a population consist of a date of birth and a date of death of other causes than colorectal cancer.

Subsequently the natural history part of MISCAN-Colon simulates colorectal cancer histories (natural histories in the absence of screening or surveillance) for each individual life history separately. We based our natural history model on the adenoma–carcinoma sequence described by Morson and colleagues[42,43], and expanded by Vogelstein et al.[44] to incorporate genetic changes associated with progression from adenoma to carcinoma. Alternative pathways, such as the Micro Satellite Instability (MSI) pathway and the MSI low pathway, can be modelled as special variants of the adenoma–carcinoma sequence[45].

Table 1 Classification of the model parameters

Parameters that are directly estimated from available data	Parameters for which no or only limited data are available	Parameters that are varied to fit reference data (calibrated)
Demography	Duration distribution in preclinical states	Probability for an adenoma to be progressive
Distribution of lesions over the colon and rectum	Transition probabilities from preclinical non-invasive states	Individual risk index
Survival after clinical diagnosis	Correlation between durations in subsequent states	Incidence rate of adenomas
Sensitivity, specificity and reach of screening tests	Dependency of test outcomes	Transition probabilities from preclinical invasive states to clinical states

The classification of the model parameters by availability of evidence-based studies is given in Table 1. Whenever possible the assumptions of the MISCAN-Colon model are based on evidence from the literature; however, in some cases expert opinion was used to inform the model. The model format was presented at two meetings at the United States National Cancer Institute with experts in the field of colorectal cancer. Adenomas are generated according to a personal risk index and an age-specific incidence rate, resulting in no adenomas for most people and one or more adenomas for others. The disease stages that are distinguished in the modeled adenoma–carcinoma sequence are shown in Figure 1.

It is assumed that adenomas are either non-progressive and will never develop into cancer in a lifetime, or progressive and are destined to develop into colorectal cancer. The average duration between incidence of a progressive adenoma and clinical diagnosis of cancer is assumed to be 20 years. The duration between adenoma incidence and preclinical colorectal cancer is assumed to be exponentially distributed with a mean of 16.4 years, while the duration of preclinical cancer is exponentially distributed with a mean of 3.6 years. It is assumed that polypectomy completely prevents growth of the polyp into cancer. Adenoma size is highly correlated with adenoma histology and high-grade dysplasia[46]. At this time the MISCAN model includes adenoma size but does not include a separate component for tubular, tubulovillous, and villous histology.

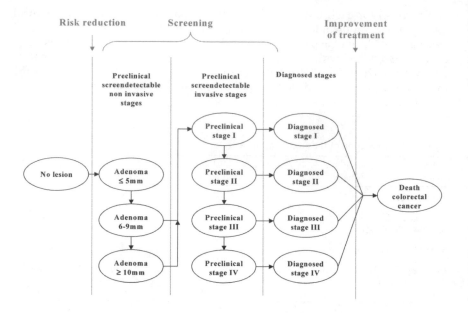

Figure 1   Natural history and possible interventions in MISCAN-Colon

If all individuals have equal risk for adenomas, i.e. adenomas are randomly distributed over the population, the resulting adenoma multiplicity is Poisson distributed. However, autopsy studies show variation larger than Poisson[47], probably because of variation in genetic and environmental factors. The model accounts for the heterogeneity in adenoma multiplicity by drawing a risk index for each individual. The individual adenoma incidence rate is equal to the individual risk index multiplied by the age-specific adenoma incidence rate. This risk index is drawn from a gamma distribution with mean 1 and a variance of 2, which is chosen to fit the multiplicity distribution of adenomas in autopsy studies[48]. The probability that a new adenoma is progressive is age-dependent but does not depend on the individual risk index. The age-specific adenoma incidence and the probability that an adenoma is progressive is chosen to fit observed US cancer incidence in 1978 before the introduction of screening and prevalence of adenomas in autopsy and colonoscopy studies[47,49-52].

In a parallel manner the MISCAN-Colon model also generates the same birth cohorts with the natural history as described above, but now with the effect of interventions such a screening or surveillance on the eventual outcome of colorectal cancer incidence or death. The effect of the intervention is derived from the difference in the outcomes from the natural history model and from the intervention model.

Although the MISCAN-Colon model was originally designed for evaluation of population-based screening in an asymptomatic population[40] it can also be used to simulate surveillance after polypectomy in patients who have had adenomas removed as in the NPS. The output of the model consists of the adenoma and cancer detection rates at initial and surveillance colonoscopy and the effect of initial and surveillance colonoscopy on cancer incidence and mortality. The main assumptions are given in Table 2 for the natural history and intervention effects, as well as the specific assumptions to simulate the NPS cohort of adenoma patients. Furthermore MISCAN-Colon is calibrated to:

- pre-screening (1975–1979) SEER incidence rates by age, location, gender and race;

- pre-screening adenoma prevalence by age and gender, assessed from autopsy studies;

- pre-screening stage distribution by age, location, gender and race.

THE NPS

The NPS was a randomized controlled trial of colonoscopic surveillance in patients who have had at least one adenoma removed[33]. All patients referred for colonoscopy or polypectomy between November 1980 and February 1990 in seven participating centres who did not have a family or personal history of familial polyposis, inflammatory bowel disease, or a personal history of polypectomy or colorectal cancer, were eligible for enrollment in the study. A total of 9112 subjects referred for colonoscopy were candidates for the study. Of these patients, 6480 were not eligible for the NPS because they did not meet the eligibility criteria of having one or more adenomatous polyps. A total of 4763 were excluded because no polyps were found. Other excluded subjects were 776 with non-adenomatous polyps only, 549 with colorectal cancer, 149 with inflammatory bowel disease or other conditions, and 35 with a sessile adenoma with a base larger than 3 cm. If the first colonoscopy was incomplete, a repeat colonoscopy was scheduled. The colon had to be cleared after three examinations and within 3 months for the patient to be part of the study; 208 patients with incomplete initial examinations were excluded. Of the included patients, 13% had more than one colonoscopy. Of the 2632 eligible patients, 1214 patients were eligible but did not choose to participate and 1418 patients consented to participate and were randomized to one of two arms. The eligible but non-randomized and the eligible randomized adenoma patients had similar characteristics[33]. All detected polyps were removed and a surveillance colonoscopy was offered to the randomized patients in arm A at 1, 3 and 6 years after initial colonoscopy and in arm B at 3 and 6 years after initial colonoscopy. If the colon was not cleared with high confidence at surveillance colonoscopy, the patient was scheduled for repeat colonoscopy. Mean follow-up time was 5.9 years. Five cancers were found during the trial (CI 1.6–11.7) (two in arm A and three in arm B), while 21 were expected based on the US population with the same age and sex distribution[8], and 43–48 were expected based on a comparison with two polyp-bearing cohorts without

Table 2 Main assumptions in the expert MISCAN-Colon model, established in expert meetings at the National Cancer Institute in 1996 and 1997

Parameter	Value	Based on
Adenoma incidence in general population	Age dependent: 40–49 years: 0.9% per year 50–59 years: 1.9% per year 60–69 years: 3.3% per year 70–79 years: 2.6% per year	Adenoma prevalence in autopsy and colonoscopy studies of 15% in age group 50–59 to 33% in age group 70+[47,49-52] and cancer incidence in SEER registry in 1978
Adenoma incidence in NPS population*	Age dependent: 40–49 years: 2.9% per year 50–59 years: 6.1% per year 60–69 years: 7.4% per year 70–79 years: 5.9% per year	Resulting from the assumed adenoma incidence in the general population and the construction of the NPS population
Duration distributions in preclinical stages	Exponential	Expert opinion, other cancer models[53-55]
Mean duration of non-progressive adenomas	Lifelong	Expert opinion
Mean duration of progressive adenomas	16.4 years	Expert opinion
Mean duration of preclinical cancer	3.6 years	Cancer detection rate at first screening and background cancer incidence in FOBT trials[56,57]
Probability to develop cancer from removed adenoma	0%	Expert opinion
Probability that a new adenoma is progressive	Dependent on age at onset: 0–65 years: 14% 65–100 years: linearly increasing from 14% to 96%	Adenoma prevalence in autopsy and colonoscopy studies of 15% in age group 50–59 to 33% in age group 70+[47,49-52], cancer incidence in SEER registry in 1978

Table 2 (continued)

Parameter	Value	Based on
Distribution of risk for adenomas over the general population	Gamma distributed, mean 1, variance 2	Multiplicity distribution of adenomas in autopsy studies[47]
Sensitivity of fictitious screening test	Adenoma ≤5 mm: 15% Adenoma 6–9 mm: 28% Adenoma 10+ mm: 99% Cancer: 100%	Adenoma size at initial polypectomy of all patients included in the NPS
Sensitivity of initial and surveillance colonoscopic examination	Adenoma ≤5 mm: 80% Adenoma 6–9 mm: 85% Adenoma 10+ mm: 95% Cancer: 95%	Back-to-back colonoscopy studies[58-60]
Reach of initial and surveillance colonoscopic examination	100%	NPS design[33]

*This is not an explicit assumption, but a consequence of the assumptions about adenoma incidence in the general population and the construction of the simulated NPS population.

intervention[10,61]. All five cancers were asymptomatic malignant adenomas detected at surveillance colonoscopy.

MISCAN SIMULATION OF THE NPS COHORT

We use the MISCAN-Colon microsimulation model to simulate a population of adenoma patients of the same age, sex and baseline adenoma characteristics of the NPS. The participants in the NPS had adenomas diagnosed and removed. The MISCAN-Colon model is adapted to this situation by applying a fictitious screening test to the general population to select individuals with adenomas detected at diagnostic colonoscopy. The fictitious screening test can be regarded as a combination of faecal occult blood test (FOBT) and sigmoidoscopy. These individuals constituted the simulated trial population. Figure 2 shows how the simulated NPS population was constructed. As in the NPS, simulated individuals with colorectal cancer diagnosed at the diagnostic colonoscopy were excluded from the trial population. The sensitivity of the fictitious screening test was adjusted to reproduce the age distribution, the distribution of adenomas over the distal and proximal colon, and the size and multiplicity distribution of adenomas at initial polypectomy in the NPS.

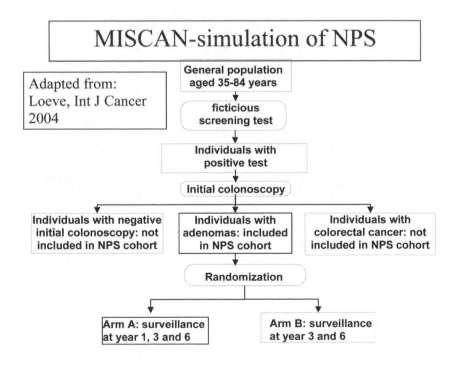

Figure 2 Simulated NPS population[62]

In the NPS, any initial or surveillance colonoscopy that was incomplete was repeated until the caecum was reached and the bowel was cleared with high confidence. For the purpose of modelling this clinical situation we define a colonoscopic examination as a series of one or more colonoscopies in a short time period of which at least one reaches the caecum and the examination is considered to be of high confidence. In the model it is assumed that all initial and surveillance colonoscopic examinations consist of one colonoscopy and that the reach of the colonoscopy is 100%, i.e. the complete bowel is visualized so that subsequently none of the patients need to undergo a second colonoscopy. Sensitivity of the initial and surveillance colonoscopic examinations is based on tandem studies of colonoscopy and increases from 80% for adenomas $\leqslant 5$ mm to 95% for preclinical cancer[58-60]. Specific assumptions for the MISCAN model to reflect the NPS population are included in Table 2. The NPS surveillance schema and the observed compliance rates per arm and surveillance round are applied to the simulated trial population.

MODEL VALIDATION

An essential component of developing the microsimulation model is to compare the model's prediction of observed rates with the actual data. This is essential for parameters that cannot be measured directly, such as sojourn times and transition rates of adenomas and cancers. In validation studies we simulate real screening and surveillance trials. When the model estimates closely correspond to the observed data, then the tested assumptions of the model are validated. Where there are discrepancies, possible external reasons are analysed. If these are insufficient, the assumptions of the model are reviewed to understand where the model needs to be modified. We assess which parameter value combinations most closely reproduce the data. This is done by calibrating with an adapted version of the Nelder and Mead Simplex method[63,64]. If there is no such combination, the model structure is adapted in a plausible way to one that can explain the data. This whole process provides for a better understanding of the disease and how it is affected by screening, and in a better-informed microsimulation model.

RESULTS

The MISCAN-Colon model simulations produced an adenoma population similar to the observed NPS with respect to the baseline characteristics of the NPS subjects (Table 3)[62]. However, the surveillance results of the simulated data estimated more colorectal cancers and fewer adenomas than observed in the NPS surveillance data. The simulated data estimated a colorectal cancer incidence rate of 1.5 per 1000 person-years in comparison to the observed rate of 0.6 per 1000 person-years. Also the simulated data estimated an 18% adenoma detection rate at the surveillance examinations which was considerably lower than the observed 27% over the 3-year surveillance.

Table 3 Characteristics at initial polypectomy of all patients and their adenomatous polyps included in the NPS, as observed in the NPS and as simulated in the expert MISCAN-Colon model (n = 1418)

Characteristic	Observed (%)	Simulated (%)
Age (years)		
<50	13	11
50–59	28	27
60–69	39	40
70–79	18	20
80+	2	3
Adenoma size*		
≤5 mm	27	27
6–9 mm	18	17
≥10 mm	55	56
No. of adenomas*		
1	57	61
2	22	23
≥3	20	16
Site of largest adenoma*		
Distal colon	64	61
Proximal colon	36	39

*Forty-four patients with polyps classified as adenomas by the local pathologist were classified as non-adenomas by the review pathologists and were excluded from the NPS cohort simulated in this modelling study (n = 1374).

We considered seven different models with the assumptions modified to increase the simulated number of adenomas and decrease the number of colorectal cancers detected at surveillance so that the simulated data were more consistent with the observed values. Three models modified assumptions to raise the adenoma detection rate at surveillance. These included lowering the adenoma sensitivity to 60%, increasing the adenoma incidence, and increasing the adenoma incidence plus assuming regression of adenomas. Two models modified assumptions with the intent to reduce the cancer incidence rate. These included assuming a model with no fast-growing adenomas and a constant duration of 20 years for sojourn time and another model with 100% sensitivity for colonoscopic detection of colorectal cancer. There were two models designed to both reduce the cancer incidence and increase the adenoma detection rate. These included a model assuming no fast-growing adenomas, a high adenoma incidence and spontaneous regression; and another model with high cancer sensitivity, high adenoma incidence and spontaneous regression. All three models that included an assumption that adenomas could regress significantly improved the original model fit. The results of the three regression models, as well as the observed and expert model estimates, are given in Table 4.

Table 4 Cancer incidence rate and proportion of surveillance examinations with adenomas as observed in the NFS population and as simulated with the expert MISCAN-Colon model and several model variants

	Cancer rate per 1000 person-years			Proportion of surveillance examinations with adenomas				Deviance
	Surveillance detected	Interval detected	All	Arm A year 1	Arm A year 3	Arm B year 3	All	
Observed	0.6	0.0	0.6*	0.28	0.22	0.32	0.27**	
Expert MISCAN-Colon assumptions	0.6	0.9	1.5	0.17	0.13	0.25	0.18	84
Model assumptions including regression of adenomas								
High adenoma incidence and spontaneous regression	0.5	0.7	1.1	0.21	0.25	0.34	0.26	24
No fast-growing adenomas, high adenoma incidence and spontaneous regression	0.2	0.2	0.4	0.21	0.25	0.35	0.27	27
High cancer sensitivity, high adenoma incidence and spontaneous regression	0.4	0.6	1.0	0.22	0.25	0.34	0.26	23

*95% Confidence interval 0.2–1.4.

**95% Confidence interval 0.25–0.30.

DISCUSSION

The MISCAN-Colon model successfully simulated the baseline and surveillance outcomes of the NPS of adenoma patients under colonoscopic surveillance. However, in developing the MISCAN-Colon modelling for the NPS it was necessary to make the model assumption that adenomas can regress in order to obtain a good match between the simulated and observed results. Although adenoma regression has not been included as a central component of the adenoma–carcinoma sequence, there have been previous findings in short-term studies that adenomas may disappear or regress in size[65-67] and that the adenoma prevalence does not noticeably increase after age 70[47,49-52]. Adenoma regression was also reported to a slight degree in the placebo arm of a randomized controlled trial of celecoxib in familial adenomatous polyposis[68]. These clinical findings support a role for adenoma regression in the adenoma–carcinoma sequence. The MISCAN model results are consistent with a role for adenoma regression. The cost-effectiveness of screening and surveillance for colorectal cancer can be assessed with this simulated cohort when regression could remove adenomas without the interventions of screening or surveillance.

The MISCAN-Colon simulated model for the NPS can now be used to consider extensions of the NPS to clinical situations which were not directly observed in the study, but which are pertinent for effective and efficient use of colonoscopic surveillance. For example we can now use microsimulation modelling to discover the separate effects of initial and surveillance colonoscopies. Furthermore we can address whether all patients require 3-year surveillance or whether the surveillance colonoscopies could be lengthened for lower-risk patients. The microsimulation methodology could also provide an assessment of whether virtual colonoscopy could be used for the screening and surveillance for lower-risk patients without diminishing the incidence reduction achieved.

The NPS demonstrated that colonoscopic polypectomy and surveillance were associated with a 76–90% reduction in colorectal cancer incidence[8]. This large reduction was achieved with all NPS patients having initial colonoscopy and surveillance colonoscopy. It is important to assess whether the incidence reduction was due to the initial colonoscopy, the surveillance colonoscopy, or to both. Although we did not directly observe the NPS cohort in this manner, we can use the MISCAN-Colon model to assess the NPS simulated cohort under three different scenarios (below) to assess the separate effects of the initial and surveillance colonoscopies:

1. no initial and no surveillance colonoscopies;

2. initial colonoscopy intervention but no surveillance;

3. initial colonoscopy and surveillance colonoscopies.

The simulated results will provide an assessment of the number of colorectal cancers that would have developed with no intervention at baseline or surveillance, with baseline colonoscopy only, and with both baseline and surveillance interventions. The overall incidence reduction will be estimated as difference in the number of colorectal cancers with neither initial nor surveillance colonoscopy compared to the number of colorectal cancers with both initial and surveillance colonoscopies. The impact of the surveillance colonoscopy is the reduction in the number of colorectal cancers with initial colonoscopy only versus the number of colorectal cancers in those with initial and surveillance colonoscopy. The simulation modelling can extend the surveillance interval assessment beyond the mean follow-up of 5.9 years and provide an assessment of the length of time that the initial or surveillance colonoscopies provides a reduction in colorectal cancer risk.

In the NPS, all five colorectal cancers were asymptomatic and detected at surveillance colonoscopies in 1418 patients. There were no colorectal cancers detected until 3 years after the initial colonoscopy. These findings are in contrast to those reported by Robertson et al.[31] in combining data from three chemoprevention studies in which 19 colorectal cancers were detected in 2915 patients. Of the 19 cancers 15 (79%) were detected during a surveillance colonoscopy and considered asymptomatic; four cancers were detected due to symptoms. There were five cancers detected within 1 year of the initial colonoscopy. The Polyp Prevention Trial, a randomized controlled trial of healthy diet (low fat, high fibre, high fruit and vegetable diet) compared to usual-care diet in adenoma patients, had 13 colorectal cancers detected in 2079 patients. There were eight asymptomatic cancers detected at surveillance colonoscopies and five cancers detected within 1 year of the initial colonoscopy[69]. These results from the chemoprevention studies might suggest that the initial colonoscopy does not provide adequate protection against colorectal cancer. However, the patient accrual for the NPS and the chemoprevention studies differed, and the method of accrual probably affected the findings within the first year of the respective studies. Those accrued to the NPS were ascertained prospectively at the initial colonoscopy and received a study protocol colonoscopy which reached the caecum and had rigorous clearing of the bowel of all polyps no matter how small. In contrast the chemoprevention studies ascertained the adenoma patients retrospectively after the adenoma diagnosis and the patient's initial colonoscopy was not according to a study protocol; it is therefore more likely that some colorectal cancers were missed at the initial colonoscopy. Loeve et al.[37] used a large national Dutch pathology database on patients with adenomas removed to assess colorectal cancer incidence after adenoma removal; 78 473 adenoma patients were followed for a mean of 4.5 years after adenoma removal. Although the recommendation was that all adenomas should be removed, and the patient should have a full colonoscopy, whether this was done was not noted in the database. Consequently these data probably include some patients with incomplete clearing of the colon after diagnosis of at least one adenoma. Loeve et al. showed that there was an excess risk of colorectal cancer up to 5 years after the diagnosis of the adenoma. These data suggest that those with adenomas which are not completely removed, or without further assessment of accompanying adenomas or colorectal cancers, have an elevated risk for colorectal cancer. The MISCAN-Colon model can be used to simulate the impact of a quality initial colonoscopy on subsequent colorectal cancer risk.

The results from this simulation would facilitate quantifying the effect of high-quality colonoscopy[70].

As more patients are screened for colorectal cancer, more adenomas are detected and the patients placed in colonoscopic surveillance programmes. The resources required for endoscopic surveillance are mounting in the United States. The MISCAN modelling of the NPS cohort can also address whether there are some adenoma patients who are not at increased risk for subsequent colorectal cancer, provided they had received a high-quality initial colonoscopy with removal of all adenomas detected. Atkin et al.[10] studied the colon cancer incidence in a cohort of rectosigmoid adenoma patients whose rectosigmoid adenomas were removed but with no further intervention in the rest of the colon. Based on the rectosigmoid cohort they showed that those with a single small (< 1.0 cm) tubular adenoma had a 50% lower risk of colon cancer than the general population, but that those with tubulovillous, villous, or adenomas of size ⩾1.0 cm had a 2.9-fold increased risk compared with the general population. The NPS has reported that patients with three or more adenomas at baseline, or those patients age 60 or older and with a family history of colorectal cancer, have a 6-fold increased risk for advanced adenomas at surveillance colonoscopy[36]. Multiplicity has also been reported as a risk factor for subsequent advanced adenomas in randomized controlled trials of chemoprevention as well as in historical prospective registry studies[10,25,29,31].

Adenoma size has also been cited as a risk factor for subsequent advanced adenomas[10,15,27–29,35]. However, the NPS did not find adenoma size to be the strongest predictor for subsequent advanced adenomas. It can be hypothesized that with the rigorous protocol colonoscopy examination of the NPS, large polyps were completely removed, whereas in the more retrospective accrual of adenoma patients, there was incomplete removal of some of the larger adenomas. The MISCAN-Colon model can be used to simulate an adenoma cohort with and without complete removal of the larger adenomas to ascertain the effect of incomplete removal on subsequent colorectal cancer risk. The current assumption in the MISCAN-Colon model for simulating the NPS data is that all detected adenomas are completely removed and, once removed, the adenoma does not become a colorectal cancer.

The MISCAN-Colon model can also be used to further assess which patient or adenoma characteristics are the best predictors of subsequent risk and what surveillance intervals for the lower- and the higher-risk patients provides the lowest colorectal cancer rates with the fewest colonoscopies. We will consider these scenarios by patient characteristics for multiplicity (one, two, or three or more adenomas) and the size (small (⩽0.5 cm), medium (0.6–0.9 cm), or large ⩾1.0 cm)) of the adenomas at initial colonoscopy. The groupings by patient characteristic will include: one small (⩽0.5 cm) adenoma; two small adenomas or one or two medium-size adenomas; one or two large adenomas but fewer than three adenomas; three or more adenomas of any size; and a combined grouping of three or more adenomas or one or more large adenomas. In addition the timing of the surveillance colonoscopies will be varied for 3, 6, or 10 years post-polypectomy by the different patient groups.

We will also consider whether virtual colonoscopy has a role in surveillance for lower-risk adenoma patients. Virtual colonoscopy has low sensitivity for adenomas of size $\leqslant 0.5$ cm[71]. We can use the NPS simulated results for the single small adenoma for the three scenarios of no initial or surveillance colonoscopies, initial colonoscopy only, and initial and surveillance colonoscopy to assess the effect of virtual colonoscopy's low sensitivity for small adenomas.

In conclusion, microsimulation modelling provides a valuable tool to assess the impact of colonoscopy screening and surveillance and guidance in the best methods to prevent colorectal cancers. Even more importantly, this tool can be used to quantify the benefits of reduced colorectal cancer rates relative to the risks of colonoscopy perforation and can suggest a balance of risks and benefits relative to the patient's risk for subsequent advanced adenomas. The simulation modelling will provide a measure for the benefit of extending the surveillance intervals for those at lower risk and the benefit of surveillance colonoscopy for those in higher-risk group.

References

1. Cancer Facts and Figures: American Cancer Society, 2005.
2. Hardcastle JD, Chamberlain JO, Robinson MH et al. Randomised controlled trial of faecal-occult-blood screening for colorectal cancer. Lancet. 1996;348:1472–7.
3. Kronborg O, Fenger C, Olsen J, Jorgensen OD, Sondergaard O. Randomised study of screening for colorectal cancer with faecal-occult-blood test. Lancet. 1996;348:1467–71.
4. Mandel JS, Bond JH, Church TR et al. Reducing mortality from colorectal cancer by screening for fecal occult blood. Minnesota Colon Cancer Control Study. N Engl J Med. 1993;328:1365–71.
5. Lieberman DA, Weiss DG, Bond JH, Ahnen DJ, Garewal H, Chejfec G. Use of colonoscopy to screen asymptomatic adults for colorectal cancer. Veterans Affairs Cooperative Study Group 380. N Engl J Med. 2000;343:162–8.
6. Imperiale TF, Wagner DR, Lin CY, Larkin GN, Rogge JD, Ransohoff DF. Risk of advanced proximal neoplasms in asymptomatic adults according to the distal colorectal findings. N Engl J Med. 2000;343:169–74.
7. Schoenfeld P, Cash B, Flood A et al. Colonoscopic screening of average-risk women for colorectal neoplasia. N Engl J Med. 2005;352:2061–8.
8. Winawer SJ, Zauber AG, Ho MN et al. Prevention of colorectal cancer by colonoscopic polypectomy. The National Polyp Study Workgroup. N Engl J Med. 1993;329:1977–81.
9. Citarda F, Tomaselli G, Capocaccia R, Barcherini S, Crespi M. Efficacy in standard clinical practice of colonoscopic polypectomy in reducing colorectal cancer incidence. Gut. 2001; 48:812–15.
10. Atkin WS, Morson BC, Cuzick J. Long-term risk of colorectal cancer after excision of rectosigmoid adenomas. N Engl J Med. 1992;326:658–62.
11. Thiis-Evensen E, Hoff GS, Sauar J, Langmark F, Majak BM, Vatn MH. Population-based surveillance by colonoscopy: effect on the incidence of colorectal cancer. Telemark Polyp Study I. Scand J Gastroenterol. 1999;34:414–20.
12. Selby JV, Friedman GD, Quesenberry CP Jr, Weiss NS. A case–control study of screening sigmoidoscopy and mortality from colorectal cancer. N Engl J Med. 1992;326:653–7.
13. Newcomb PA, Norfleet RG, Storer BE, Surawicz TS, Marcus PM. Screening sigmoidoscopy and colorectal cancer mortality. J Natl Cancer Inst. 1992;84:1572–5.
14. Newcomb PA, Storer BE, Morimoto LM, Templeton A, Potter JD. Long-term efficacy of sigmoidoscopy in the reduction of colorectal cancer incidence. J Natl Cancer Inst. 2003;95: 622–5.
15. Bertario L, Russo A, Sala P et al. Predictors of metachronous colorectal neoplasms in sporadic adenoma patients. Int J Cancer. 2003;105:82–7.
16. Winawer S, Fletcher R, Rex D et al. Colorectal cancer screening and surveillance: clinical guidelines and rationale – update based on new evidence. Gastroenterology. 2003;124:544–60.

17. Smith RA, von Eschenbach AC, Wender R et al. American Cancer Society guidelines for the early detection of cancer: update of early detection guidelines for prostate, colorectal, and endometrial cancers. Also: update 2001 – testing for early lung cancer detection. Cancer J Clin. 2001;51:38–75;77–80.
18. Winawer SJ, Fletcher RH, Miller L et al. Colorectal cancer screening: clinical guidelines and rationale. Gastroenterology. 1997;112:594–642.
19. Byers BL, Rothenberger D, Dodd GD, Smith RA. American Cancer Society guidelines for screening and surveillance for early detection of colorectal polyps and cancer: update 1997. Cancer J Clin. 1997;47:154–60.
20. Vijan S, Inadomi J, Hayward RA, Hofer TP, Fendrick AM. Projections of demand and capacity for colonoscopy related to increasing rates of colorectal cancer screening in the United States. Aliment Pharmacol Ther. 2004;20:507–15.
21. Ladabaum U, Song K. Projected national impact of colorectal cancer screening on clinical and economic outcomes and health services demand. Gastroenterology. 2005;129:1151–62.
22. Seeff LC, Tangka FK. Can we predict the outcomes of national colorectal cancer screening and can predictions help us plan? Gastroenterology. 2005;129:1339–42.
23. Winawer SJ, Zauber AG, Fletcher RH et al. Post-polypectomy surveillance guidelines: a consensus update by the US Multi-Society Task Force on colorectal cancer and the American Cancer Society. Gastroenterology. 2006;130 (In press).
24. Avidan B, Sonnenberg A, Schnell TG, Leya J, Metz A, Sontag SJ. New occurrence and recurrence of neoplasms within 5 years of a screening colonoscopy. Am J Gastroenterol. 2002;97:1524–9.
25. Bonithon-Kopp C, Piard F, Fenger C et al. Colorectal adenoma characteristics as predictors of recurrence. Dis Colon Rectum. 2004;47:323–33.
26. Fossi S, Bazzoli F, Ricciardiello L et al. Incidence and recurrence rates of colorectal adenomas in first-degree asymptomatic relatives of patients with colon cancer. Am J Gastroenterol. 2001;96:1601–4.
27. Lieberman DA, Weiss DG. 5-year surveillance of patients with adenomas or colorectal cancer at screening colonoscopy: results from the VA Cooperative Study no. 380. Gastroenterology. 2004;126:A22.
28. Martinez ME, Sampliner R, Marshall JR, Bhattacharyya AK, Reid ME, Alberts DS. Adenoma characteristics as risk factors for recurrence of advanced adenomas. Gastroenterology. 2001;120:1077–83.
29. Noshirwani KC, van Stolk RU, Rybicki LA, Beck GJ. Adenoma size and number are predictive of adenoma recurrence: implications for surveillance colonoscopy. Gastrointest Endosc. 2000;51:433–7.
30. Nusko G, Mansmann U, Kirchner T, Hahn EG. Risk related surveillance following colorectal polypectomy. Gut. 2002;51:424–8.
31. Robertson DJ, Greenberg ER, Beach M et al. Colorectal cancer in patients under close colonoscopic surveillance. Gastroenterology. 2005;129:34–41.
32. van Stolk RU, Beck GJ, Baron JA, Haile R, Summers R. Adenoma characteristics at first colonoscopy as predictors of adenoma recurrence and characteristics at follow-up. Polyp Prevention Study Group. Gastroenterology. 1998;115:13–18.
33. Winawer SJ, Zauber AG, O'Brien MJ et al. Randomized comparison of surveillance intervals after colonoscopic removal of newly diagnosed adenomatous polyps. National Polyp Study Workgroup. N Engl J Med. 1993;328:901–6.
34. Yamaji Y, Mitsushima T, Ikuma H et al. Incidence and recurrence rates of colorectal adenomas estimated by annually repeated colonoscopies on asymptomatic Japanese. Gut. 2004;53:568–72.
35. Yang G, Zheng W, Sun QR et al. Pathologic features of initial adenomas as predictors for metachronous adenomas of the rectum. J Natl Cancer Inst. 1998;90:1661–5.
36. Zauber AG, Winawer SJ, Bond J et al. Can surveillance intervals be lengthened following colonoscopic polypectomy? Gastroenterology. 1997;112:A50.
37. Loeve F, van Ballegooijen M, Boer R, Kuipers EJ, Habbema JD. Colorectal cancer risk in adenoma patients: a nation-wide study. Int J Cancer. 2004;111:147–51.
38. Loeve F, Boer R, van Oortmarssen GJ, van Ballegooijen M, Habbema JDF. The MISCAN-Colon simulation model for the evaluation of colorectal cancer screening. Comput Biomed Res. 1999;32:13–33.

39. Loeve F, Boer R, Ballegooijen Mv, Oortmarssen GJv, Habbema JDF. Final Report MISCAN-Colon Microsimulation Model for Colorectal Cancer. Report to the NCI, Project No. N01.CN55186. Rotterdam: Department of Public Health, Erasmus University, 1998.
40. Loeve F, Brown ML, Boer R, van Ballegooijen M, van Oortmarssen GJ, Habbema JD. Endoscopic colorectal cancer screening: a cost-saving analysis. J Natl Cancer Inst. 2000;92: 557–63.
41. Vogelaar I, van Ballegooijen M, Zauber AG. Department of Public Health, Erasmus MC. Model Profiler of the MISCAN-Colon microsimulation model for colorectal cancer, 2004.
42. Morson B. The polyp–cancer sequence in the large bowel. Proc R Soc Med. 1974;67:451–7.
43. Muto T, Bussey H, Morson BC. The evolution of cancer of the colon and rectum. Cancer. 1975;36:2251–70.
44. Vogelstein B, Fearon ER, Hamilton SR et al. Genetic alterations during colorectal-tumor development. N Engl J Med. 1988;319:525–32.
45. O'Brien MJ, Yang S, Clebanoff JL et al. Hyperplastic (serrated) polyps of the colorectum: relationship of CpG island methylator phenotype and K-ras mutation to location and histologic subtype. Am J Surg Pathol. 2004;28:423–34.
46. O'Brien MJ, Winawer SJ, Zauber AG et al. The National Polyp Study. Patient and polyp characteristics associated with high-grade dysplasia in colorectal adenomas. Gastroenterology. 1990;98:371–9.
47. Koretz RL. Malignant polyps: are they sheep in wolves' clothing? Ann Intern Med. 1993; 118:63–8.
48. Diggle PJ, Liang K, Zeger SL. Analysis of Longitudinal Data. Oxford: Oxford Science Publications, Clarendon Press, 1994.
49. Johnson DA, Gurney MS, Volpe RJ et al. A prospective study of the prevalence of colonic neoplasms in asymptomatic patients with an age-related risk. Am J Gastroenterol. 1990; 85:969–74.
50. DiSario JA, Foutch PG, Mai HD, Pardy K, Manne RK. Prevalence and malignant potential of colorectal polyps in asymptomatic, average-risk men. Am J Gastroenterol. 1991;86:941–5.
51. Lieberman DA, Smith FW. Screening for colon malignancy with colonoscopy. Am J Gastroenterol. 1991;86:946–51.
52. Rex DK, Lehman GA, Hawes RH, Ulbright TM, Smith JJ. Screening colonoscopy in asymptomatic average-risk persons with negative fecal occult blood tests. Gastroenterology. 1991;100:64–7.
53. Walter SD, Day NE. Estimation of the duration of a pre-clinical disease state using screening data. Am J Epidemiol. 1983;118:865–86.
54. Gyrd-Hansen D, Sogaard J, Kronborg O. Analysis of screening data: colorectal cancer. Int J Epidemiol. 1997;26:1172–81.
55. Launoy G, Smith TC, Duffy SW, Bouvier V. Colorectal cancer mass-screening: estimation of faecal occult blood test sensitivity, taking into account cancer mean sojourn time. Int J Cancer. 1997;73:220–4.
56. Hardcastle JD, Thomas WM, Chamberlain J et al. Randomised, controlled trial of faecal occult blood screening for colorectal cancer. Results for first 107,349 subjects. Lancet. 1989;1:1160–4.
57. Kronborg O, Fenger C, Olsen J, Bech K, Søndergaard O. Repeated screening for colorectal cancer with fecal occult blood test. A prospective randomized study at Funen, Denmark. Scand J Gastroenterol. 1989;24:599–606.
58. Hixson LJ, Fennerty MB, Sampliner RE, Garewal HS. Prospective blinded trial of the colonoscopic miss-rate of large colorectal polyps. Gastrointest Endosc. 1991;37:125–7.
59. Rex DK, Cutler CS, Lemmel GT et al. Colonoscopic miss rates of adenomas determined by back-to-back colonoscopies. Gastroenterology. 1997;112:24–8.
60. Rex DK, Rahmani EY, Haseman JH, Lemmel GT, Kaster S, Buckley JS. Relative sensitivity of colonoscopy and barium enema for detection of colorectal cancer in clinical practice. Gastroenterology. 1997;112:17–23.
61. Stryker SJ, Wolff BG, Culp CE, Libbe SD, Ilstrup DM, MacCarty RL. Natural history of untreated colonic polyps. Gastroenterology. 1987;93:1009–13.
62. Loeve F, Boer R, Zauber AG et al. National Polyp Study data: evidence for regression of adenomas. Int J Cancer. 2004;111:633–9.

63. Neddermeijer HG, Piersma N, Oortmarssen GJv, Habbema JDF, Dekker R. Comparison of response surface methodology and the Nelder and Mead simplex method for optimization in microsimulation models: Econometric Institute, 1999.

64. Nelder JA. A simplex method of function minimization. Comput J. 1965;7:308–12.

65. Knoernschild HE. Growth rate and malignant potential of colonic polyps: early results. Surg Forum. 1963;14:137–8.

66. Hoff G, Foerster A, Vatn MH, Sauar J, Larsen S. Epidemiology of polyps in the rectum and colon. Recovery and evaluation of unresected polyps 2 years after detection. Scand J Gastroenterol. 1986;21:853–62.

67. Hofstad B, Vatn MH, Andersen SN et al. Growth of colorectal polyps: redetection and evaluation of unresected polyps for a period of three years. Gut. 1996;39:449–56.

68. Steinbach G, Lynch PM, Phillips RK et al. The effect of celecoxib, a cyclooxygenase-2 inhibitor, in familial adenomatous polyposis. N Engl J Med. 2000;342:1946–52.

69. Pabby A, Schoen RE, Weissfeld JL et al. Analysis of colorectal cancer occurrence during surveillance colonoscopy in the dietary Polyp Prevention Trial. Gastrointest Endosc. 2005; 61:385–91.

70. Rex DK, Bond JH, Winawer S et al. Quality in the technical performance of colonoscopy and the continuous quality improvement process for colonoscopy: recommendations of the US Multi-Society Task Force on Colorectal Cancer. Am J Gastroenterol. 2002;97:1296–308.

71. Pickhardt PJ, Choi JR, Hwang I et al. Computed tomographic virtual colonoscopy to screen for colorectal neoplasia in asymptomatic adults. N Engl J Med. 2003;349:2191–200.

13
Differential signalling pathways of tumour-promoting and tumour-inhibiting bile acids in colonic carcinogenesis

S. KHARE, R. MUSTAFI, S. CERDA, A. FICHERA and
M. BISSONNETTE

EPIDEMIOLOGY OF BILE ACIDS AND COLON CANCER

Colorectal cancer is a leading cause of cancer-related deaths in the United States. In addition to genetic factors, dietary constituents play important roles in tumour development[1,2]. In this regard, diets high in animal fat predispose to experimental colon cancer[3]. Endogenous bile acids, secreted in response to dietary fats, are thought to contribute to this increased risk[2,4,5]. A small fraction (less than 5%) of unabsorbed bile acids enters the colon and is metabolized by colonic bacteria. In the colon, cholic acid is converted to deoxycholic acid (DCA)[1] and chenodeoxycholic acid to lithocholic acid. Epidemiological studies have suggested that these secondary bile acids promote colonic carcinogenesis[6]. In several human studies, individuals with neoplastic lesions had increased serum and/or faecal levels of secondary bile acids[4,7].

The azoxymethane (AOM) model of colon cancer recapitulates many of the clinical, histological and molecular features of human colon cancer. A tumour-promoting role for bile acids has been established in this model of colonic carcinogenesis[8-10]. A number of potential mechanisms have been proposed for bile acid-induced colonic tumour promotion, including increased oxidative damage to nucleic acids, lipids and proteins, and alterations in cell signalling, including Ras activation[11,12]. While the predominant primary bile acids are tumour promoters, we have shown that another bile acid, ursodeoxycholic acid (UDCA), is chemopreventive in AOM-induced colonic carcinogenesis[8,13]. UDCA is a relatively hydrophilic low-abundance (4%) bile acid that is widely used to treat cholestatic liver disorders[14]. In the AOM rat model our laboratory has demonstrated that UDCA possesses chemopreventive efficacy, inhibiting tumour incidence by more than 50% and preventing tumour promotion by cholic acid[8]. More recently, we showed that UDCA also suppressed the development of tumours with *ras* mutations or tumours with activated wild-type Ras[15]. In addition, UDCA limited up-regulation of cyclooxygenase-2 (Cox-2), a down-stream target of Ras in AOM-induced tumours[15,16]. Cox-2 is the rate-limiting enzyme for the biosynthesis of prostanoids and is elevated in most human and AOM-induced colonic tumours[17-19]. Prostaglandins stimulate proliferation, apoptotic resistance and angiogenesis in colonic carcinogenesis[20]. Supporting a causal role for Cox-2, cyclooxygenase inhibitors significantly reduced AOM tumour incidence[21].

Aberrant crypt foci (ACF) are the earliest identifiable putative precursors of colon cancer[22,23]. In the premalignant phase of the AOM model, UDCA inhibited the formation of ACF, whereas cholic acid promoted the growth of large ACF[16,24]. Based upon the divergent modulation induced by these bile acids in premalignancy at the ACF stage, as well as in established tumours, we hypothesized these agents might cause opposite effects on Ras effectors prior to ACF appearance. We first asked whether Ras effectors and Ras targets were altered by these bile acids in the early premalignant phase. Alterations in Ras signalling induced by bile acids at this early time point are likely to be causally related to their effects on tumourigenesis or chemoprevention. Since chemopreventive UDCA inhibited Cox-2 expression in AOM tumours, it was also of interest to examine the effect of supplementation with tumour-promoting cholic acid on Cox-2 expression in tumours. In colon cancer cells bile acids have been shown to modulate EGFR/Ras signalling[25]. In preliminary studies we found epidermal grwoth factor receptor (EGFR) signalling is up-regulated in AOM carcinogenesis[26]. To assess the potential role of EGFR in bile acid effects in tumourigenesis, we examined the effects of UDCA on EGFR activation in normal mouse colon. We also elucidated mechanisms by which these bile acids modulate EGFR/Ras signalling and Cox-2 expression *in vitro* in human HCA-7 colon cancer cells. These cells possess EGFR regulated wild-type Ras and inducible Cox-2[27].

Figure 1 Cholic acid enhances, whereas UDCA inhibits, AOM-induced Ras activation and signalling in premalignant rat colonocytes. Rats received intraperitoneal AOM (20 mg/kg) or saline and were gavaged with DMSO, cholic acid (10 mg/kg) or UDCA (50 mg/kg) twice daily for 5 days. After sacrifice premalignant colonocytes were isolated and cells pooled from three rats in each group. Control colonocytes (Ctl) were obtained from rats treated with saline (AOM vehicle) and DMSO (bile acid vehicle). Shown are representative blots of two independent experiments with comparable results. Fold activation in italics is given below each lane, and represents the means of these experiments. **A**: Ras activation and Ras expression. Cells were lysed and activated Ras (Ras-GTP) isolated by c-Raf-RBD pull-down assay. Pan-Ras in whole cell lysates and Ras-GTP were detected by Western blotting. **B**: ERK and p38 activation. ERK and p38 kinase activations were measured in whole cell lysates by Western blotting using phospho-(active) antibodies. Levels of Ras-GTP, pERK and p-p38 effector kinases in colonocytes from rats that received cholic acid or UDCA alone (no carcinogen) were comparable to control rats (data not shown). Separate samples were run for β-actin to assess comparable protein loads. **C**: Cox-2 expression. Cox-2 was immunoprecipitated from lysates and Western blotted with Cox-2 antibodies. Caco-2 cells transfected with Cox-2 cDNA served as a positive control. Cholic acid or UDCA alone did not induce Cox-2. The β-actin levels in cell lysates used for Cox-2 immunoprecipitation are shown in Figure 1B

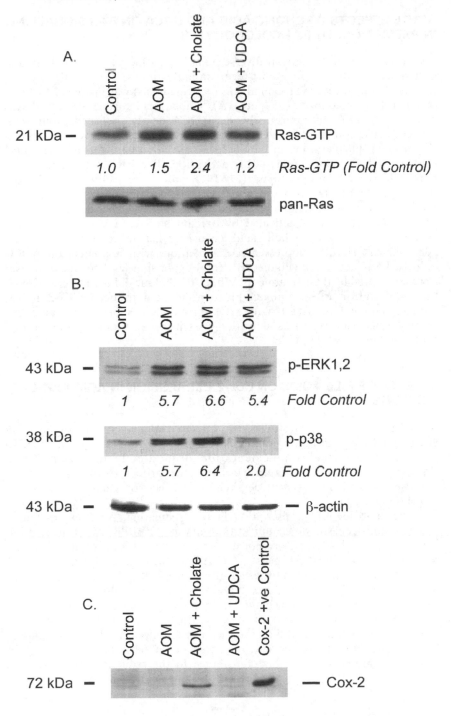

A.

21 kDa — Ras-GTP

1.0   1.5   2.4   1.2   *Ras-GTP (Fold Control)*

pan-Ras

B.

43 kDa — p-ERK1,2

1   5.7   6.6   5.4   *Fold Control*

38 kDa — p-p38

1   5.7   6.4   2.0   *Fold Control*

43 kDa — β-actin

C.

72 kDa — Cox-2

131

ACUTE EFFECTS OF CHOLIC ACID AND UDCA ON RAS SIGNALLING IN PREMALIGNANT RAT COLONOCYTES

Bile acids are known to activate diverse signalling pathways in both colonic and non-colonic cells. In our short-term animal studies, 5 days after AOM treatment constitutive GTP-bound Ras (activated Ras) was increased to 150% of control rat colonocytes (Figure 1A). Cholic acid further increased Ras activation to 240% of control, whereas UDCA nearly abolished carcinogen-induced activation. These acute treatments did not alter total Ras expression (Figure 1A). Furthermore, in the absence of AOM treatment, neither cholic acid nor UDCA alone altered Ras activation. The ERK, members of the mitogen-activated protein kinase (MAPK) family, are EGFR/Ras effectors that regulate diverse processes including physiological and neoplastic proliferation[28]. AOM treatment activated the ERK, as well as p38, another MAPK member that is activated by oxidant stresses, including alkylating agents such as AOM[29]. Cholic acid gavage further activated the ERK and p38, whereas UDCA suppressed p38 activation, with less effect on AOM-induced ERK activation (Figure 1B). Total expression levels of these kinases were not altered by these treatments. While AOM alone did not increase Cox-2, the combination of carcinogen plus cholic acid induced Cox-2 in rat premalignant colonocytes (Figure 1C). From these short-term studies we speculate that enhanced Ras activation contributes to tumour promotion by cholic acid in the AOM model.

EFFECTS OF BILE ACIDS ON Cox-2 EXPRESSION IN AOM-INDUCED TUMOURS

In agreement with earlier studies[15,16], UDCA supplementation significantly decreased Cox-2 up-regulation in AOM-induced tumours (Figure 2). In contrast, cholic acid supplementation dramatically increased Cox-2 expression in tumours (Figure 2). Thus, the proclivity of bile acids to modulate tumour development parallels their effects on Cox-2 expression in AOM tumourigenesis[8,15,16].

To begin to identify transcription factors regulating Cox-2 expression in AOM tumourigenesis, we examined tumours for C/EBPβ. This transcription factor binds to the NF-IL6 response element in the Cox-2 promoter, a *cis*-regulator of Cox-2 in HCA-7 cells[27,30]. C/EBPβ is up-regulated in human colon cancers[31]. Intriguingly, an activating isoform of C/EBPβ (M_r 45 kDa) was up-regulated in AOM tumours, and UDCA significantly inhibited this AOM-induced increased expression (Figure 3). In human adenomatous polyps, Cox-2 is initially up-regulated in macrophages, which require C/EBPβ for Cox-2 induction[32,33]. Thus, C/EBPβ appears to play an important role in regulating Cox-2 expression in colonic carcinogenesis. UDCA inhibition of C/EBPβ expression, moreover, probably contributes to the reduction in Cox-2, and thereby to the chemopreventive effects of this bile acid.

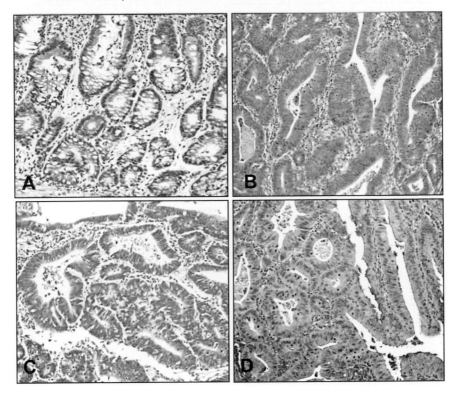

Figure 2   Cholic acid increases, whereas UDCA inhibits, Cox-2 up-regulation in AOM-induced tumours. AOM tumours were stained for Cox-2 as previously described[19]. Shown are sections from representative tumours. **A**: Control normal mucosa from an unsupplemented rat. Bile acid supplementation without AOM treatment did not alter Cox-2 expression (data not shown). **B**: AOM tumour from an unsupplemented rat. **C**: AOM tumour from a rat supplemented with UDCA. **D**: AOM tumour from a rat supplemented with cholic acid. (n = 6 tumours from the AOM alone group, 4 tumours from the AOM + cholic acid group and 6 tumours from the AOM + UDCA group). Cox-2 expression was consistently highest in the AOM + cholic acid group, intermediate in the AOM alone group, and lowest in the AOM + UDCA group. Cox-2 expression was increased in both stromal and epithelial cells

UDCA INHIBITS EGFR SIGNALLING IN NORMAL MOUSE COLON

We have recently shown in mice that AOM induces EGFR signalling, as assessed by increased phospho (active) EGFR, ErbB2, and ERK during the premalignant phase of colonic tumorigenesis[26]. Furthermore, Gefitinib, an inhibitor of EGFR, decreased ACF growth and EGFR signalling in premalignant mucosa[26]. More recently we found that Gefitinib inhibited tumour development in rats[34]. Since EGFR signalling is increased in AOM tumorigenesis, and UDCA has been shown to block EGFR/Ras/ERK signalling in DCA-treated HCT116 colon cancer cells[25], we speculated UDCA might inhibit EGFR activation in colonic carcinogenesis. To first test the ability of UDCA to inhibit EGFR activation *in vivo* we examined the effect

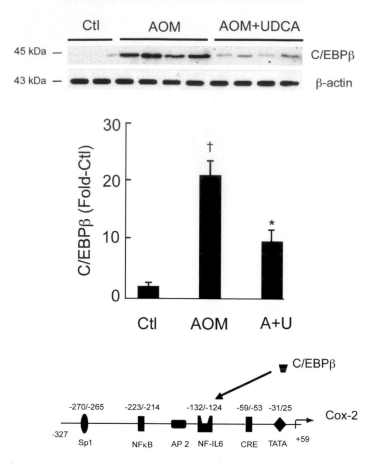

Figure 3 UDCA inhibits up-regulation of C/EBPβ in AOM-induced tumours. Colonocyte lysates from control rats and tumour lysates from rats treated with AOM alone, or rats supplemented with UDCA (A+U) were probed with C/EBPβ antibodies. Shown are means ± SD of quantitative Western blotting normalized to fold-control ($n = 4$ tumours in each group). Control colonocytes were obtained from rats that did not receive AOM. C/EBPβ expression levels in colonocytes from animals supplemented with UDCA alone (no carcinogen) were not different from controls (data not shown). [†]$p < 0.05$ compared with control; *$p < 0.05$ compared with AOM alone. *Inset:* Representative Western blot of C/EBPβ in colonocyte lysates from control rats (Ctl) or tumour cell lysates from rats given AOM alone (AOM) or AOM + UDCA. Parallel samples were run for β-actin to assess protein loads. The Cox-2 promoter with NF-IL6 response element and C/EBPβ transactivator are shown below

of UDCA on EGFR signalling in normal mouse colon. Normal mice were treated with systemic EGF and, as anticipated, growth factor signalling was activated in the colon (Figure 4A). UDCA by gavage inhibited EGFR activation and down-stream signalling *in vivo* (Figure 4A). Based on these findings in normal mouse colon and colon cancer cells, UDCA may inhibit Ras signalling in premalignancy by blocking EGFR activation.

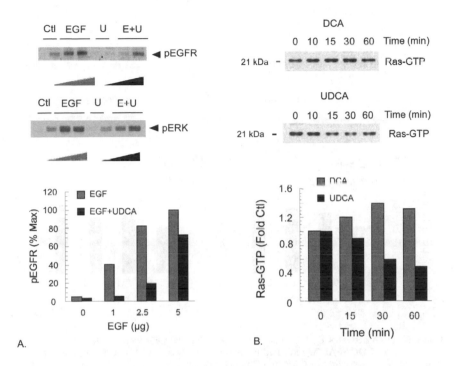

Figure 4 UDCA inhibits EGFR activation and down-stream Ras signalling *in vivo* and *in vitro*. **A**: Mice were gavaged with UDCA (50 mg/kg body weight) or vehicle (DMSO) twice daily for 5 days. Anaesthetized mice were then treated with the indicated systemic doses of EGF or vehicle (Ctl) and 5 min later colons harvested. *Upper panel*: Western blots of phospho-active EGFR (pEGFR) and phospho-active ERK (pERK). *Lower panel*: quantitative pEGFR densitometry. **B**: HCA-7 cells were treated with 100 μM DCA or UDCA and at the indicated times Ras-GTP was isolated by a Ras-GTP-pull-down assay. *Upper panel*: Ras-GTP assessed by Western blotting. *Lower panel*: quantitative densitometry

EFFECTS OF BILE ACIDS ON EGFR SIGNALLING AND Cox-2 EXPRESSION IN HUMAN HCA-7 CELLS

EGFR and Ras are important regulators of Cox-2 expression[19,27,35]. Since cholic acid increased, whereas UDCA inhibited Cox-2 expression in malignant colonocytes (Figure 2), we examined their effects in HCA-7 colon cancer cells. DCA increased Ras-GTP, whereas UDCA decreased basal Ras activity (Figure 4B). To assess the role of up-stream events, we examined the effect of DCA on EGFR signalling in these cells. As shown in Figure 5, DCA activated EGFR signalling and increased Ras-GTP. Similarly, DCA induced Cox-2 but not Cox-1 expression, whereas UDCA inhibited Cox-2 induction (Figure 6). These bile acid-induced alterations in EGFR/Ras signalling and Cox-2 induction probably play important roles in their tumour-modulating effects in colonic malignant transformation.

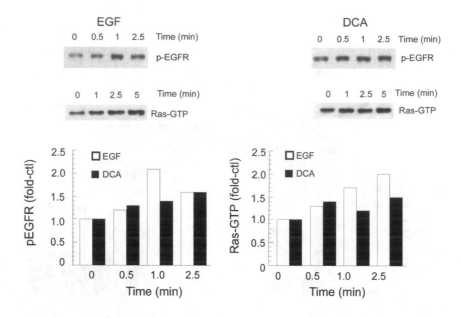

Figure 5 DCA activates EGFR signalling in HCA-7 cells. Cells were treated with 100 ng/ml EGF or 100 µM DCA. At the indicated times cells were lysed and Ras-GTP isolated by c-Raf-RBD pull-down assay and pEGFR and Ras-GTP detected by Western blotting. DCA induced EGFR activation and increased Ras-GTP in a time-dependent manner

EFFECTS OF DCA AND UDCA ON Cox-2 GENE EXPRESSION IN HCA-7 CELLS

Since Cox-2 expression is regulated at both the transcriptional and post-transcriptional levels[27], we first examined the effect of DCA on Cox-2 mRNA abundance in HCA-7 cells. Within 1 h DCA significantly up-regulated Cox-2 mRNA more than 3-fold (Figure 7A). Unlike the sustained Cox-2 protein expression induced by DCA, we found the expression of Cox-2 mRNA declined within 2 h. Preincubation with UDCA significantly inhibited DCA induction of Cox-2 mRNA in these cells (Figure 7A). Thus, similar to AOM tumours[15], UDCA suppressed Cox-2 mRNA and protein expression in HCA-7 cells (Figures 6 and 7).

To assess the contribution of altered gene transcription in the bile acid-induced changes in Cox-2 mRNA abundance, we examined the effects of DCA and UDCA on the activity of a luciferase reporter gene regulated by a Cox-2 promoter. As shown in Figure 7B, DCA caused a 3-fold increase in Cox-2 promoter activity, whereas UDCA inhibited this activation. Thus, bile acid-induced changes in Cox-2 expression in HCA-7 cells involve altered Cox-2 gene transcription and Cox-2 mRNA abundance. Cox-2 mRNA stabilization is another major mechanism regulating Cox-2 expression in many cells. Further

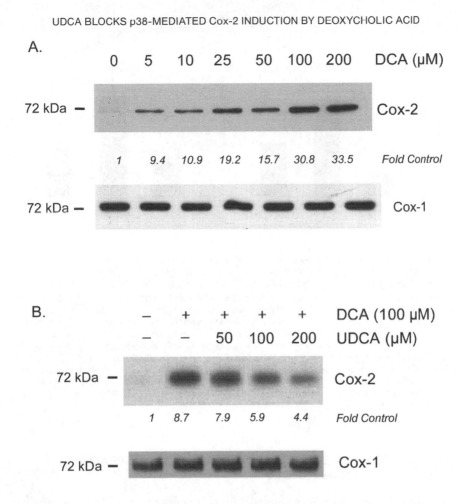

Figure 6 DCA induces Cox-2 expression in HCA-7 cells and UDCA inhibits this induction. HCA-7 cells were treated for the indicated times with the indicated bile acids. Whole cell lysates were then probed for Cox-2 expression by Western blotting. **A**: Concentration-dependence of Cox-2 induction by DCA. HCA-7 cells were treated for 6 h with the indicated concentrations of DCA (0–200 μM). **B**: UDCA inhibits Cox-2 induction by DCA. Cells were pretreated for 18 h with the indicated concentrations of UDCA and then treated with 100 μM DCA for 6 h. Separate samples were run for Cox-1 to confirm comparable protein concentrations

studies will be needed to assess whether changes in mRNA stabilization contribute to bile acid-induced alterations in mRNA abundance. We previously observed that UDCA inhibited the up-regulation of Cox-2 mRNA and protein in AOM tumours[15]. Taken together, the current results in HCA-7 cells, and our prior findings in the AOM model, suggest that this chemopreventive agent probably inhibits Cox-2 transcription in colonic carcinogenesis.

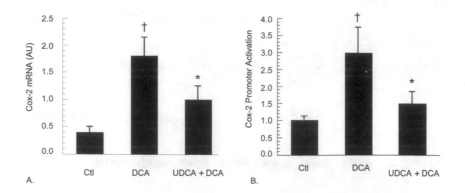

Figure 7 UDCA inhibits Cox-2 mRNA induction and Cox-2 promoter activation by DCA. **A:** Cox-2 mRNA by real-time PCR. Cells were pretreated with 100 μM UDCA or vehicle for 18 h and then 100 μM DCA or DMSO was added for 1 h. Cox-2 mRNA was determined by real-time PCR as described[15]. Cox-1 was amplified as an internal control for normalization. UDCA alone did not alter Cox-2 expression. (n = 3 independent experiments in triplicate; $^{\dagger}p < 0.05$ compared with control; $*p < 0.05$ compared with cells treated with DCA alone). **B:** Cox-2 promoter activation. Cells were transiently co-transfected with a Cox-2 promoter containing a luciferase reporter and a β-galactosidase reporter to normalize for transfection efficiency. Six hours after transfection the cells were treated with 100 μM UDCA or vehicle (DMSO) for 12 h. DCA (100 μM) or DMSO was then added for an additional 6 h. Light units were normalized to β-galactosidase activity and Cox-2 promoter activation expressed as fold of vehicle-treated cells (n = 3 independent experiments in triplicate; $^{\dagger}p < 0.05$ compared with control; $*p < 0.05$ compared with DCA alone)

DCA INDUCES Cox-2 UP-REGULATION BY A p38-DEPENDENT MECHANISM IN HCA-7 CELLS

The MAPK, ERK and p38 are important regulators of Cox-2 expression[27,36]. As shown in Figure 8, DCA activated ERK and p38 in HCA-7 cells. PD 98059, an up-stream inhibitor of ERK, blocked their activation by DCA (Figure 8A). Similarly, the p38 inhibitor SB 203580[37] blocked p38 activation induced by DCA (Figure 8B). SB 203580 abolished DCA-induced Cox-2 up-regulation, suggesting that p38 is required for Cox-2 induction by this tumour promoting bile acid (Figure 8C). Since DCA appeared to induce Cox-2 via p38, and UDCA antagonized Cox-2 induction by DCA, we examined the effects of UDCA on ERK and p38 activation by DCA. HCA-7 cell pretreatment with UDCA caused a dose-dependent decrease in DCA-induced p38 activation and Cox-2 up-regulation, but did not significantly alter pERK (Figure 9A). These results suggest that DCA induces Cox-2 via a p38-dependent pathway, whereas UDCA inhibits this induction at least in part by blocking p38 activation in HCA-7 cells. The patterns of p38 activation by DCA and p38 inhibition by UDCA in HCA-7 cells were similar to the effects of cholic acid and UDCA *in vivo* in the AOM model, i.e. cholic acid-enhanced, whereas UDCA inhibited p38 activation in premalignant colonocytes. As shown in Figure 9B, DCA, but

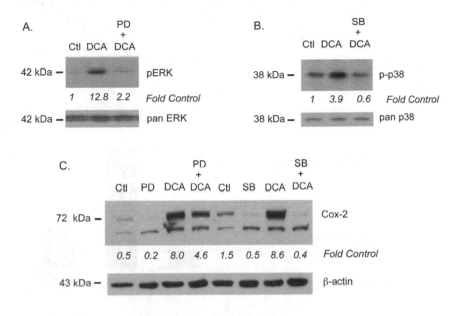

Figure 8 Cox-2 induction by DCA requires p38 signalling. HCA-7 cells were preincubated for 1 h with DMSO (vehicle, Ctl), 20 μM PD 98059 (PD), a MEK inhibitor, or 10 μM SB 203580 (SB), a p38 inhibitor. Cells were then treated with 100 μM DCA or DMSO. For kinase activations the cells were lysed 1 hr after DCA addition and whole cell lysates examined for pan and phospho-active kinase levels. For Cox-2 induction, cell incubations were continued for 18 h and Cox-2 expression determined by Western blotting. Levels of kinase activation or Cox-2 induction were expressed as fold-control and are shown below the respective blots. **A**: phospho-(active) ERK and pan-ERK; **B**: phospho-(active) p38 and pan-p38; **C**: Cox-2

not UDCA, also significantly up-regulated the Cox-2 transactivating factor C/EBPβ in these cells. In addition to expression, C/EBPβ activity is regulated by ERK and p38. Thus, the ability of DCA to increase the expression and activation of C/EBPβ would favour Cox-2 induction in colonic carcinogenesis (Figures 8 and 9). In contrast, UDCA inhibition of C/EBPβ expression and activation would limit Cox-2 induction (Figures 3 and 8).

DISCUSSION

In our studies we have demonstrated that AOM-induced carcinogenesis activated Ras, ERK and p38 prior to ACF formation. Tumour-promoting cholic acid further enhanced Ras and p38 activation, whereas chemopreventive UDCA inhibited these activations. While ERK were strongly activated at this stage of colonic premalignancy and increased by DCA, their modulation by UDCA was less striking. Cholic acid also up-regulated Cox-2 expression in premalignant and malignant colonocytes, whereas UDCA inhibited Cox-2 increases in tumours. These differential effects of bile acids on

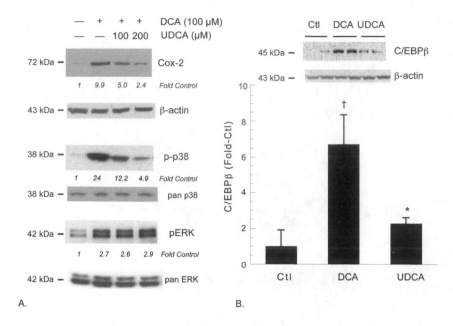

Figure 9 Effects of bile acids on p38, C/EBPβ and Cox-2 in HCA-7 cells. **A**: Cells were pre-treated for 18 h with UDCA or DMSO (vehicle), followed by 100 μM DCA or DMSO for 3 h. Cells were lysed and Cox-2, phospho-p38 and pERK determined by Western blotting. Separate samples were run for β-actin, pan-p38 and pan-ERK to confirm comparable protein loads. Results represent two independent experiments. **B**: Cells were treated with DMSO (Ctl), 100 μM DCA, or 100 μM UDCA for 4 h and C/EBPβ determined by Western blotting. Parallel samples were assessed for β-actin levels. Values were expressed as fold-control. $^{†}p < 0.05$ compared with control (DMSO); $^{*}p < 0.05$ compared with DCA

Ras signalling and Cox-2 expression *in vivo* would favour their respective tumour-promoting and tumour-inhibiting properties[8]. In studies *in vitro* in human HCA-7 colon cancer cells we found that these bile acids caused effects similar to their actions in the AOM model with respect to Ras, p38 and Cox-2.

Cox-2 plays a critical role in colonic carcinogenesis. This inducible enzyme catalyses the rate-limiting step in prostanoid biosynthesis. Cox-2 up-regulation and/or increased secretion of prostaglandins of the E2 series have been shown to enhance proliferation, inhibit apoptosis and increase invasiveness of colon cancer cells *in vitro* and *in vivo*[38]. In this chapter we showed that Cox-2 is increased in AOM tumours from rats supplemented with cholic acid, whereas Cox-2 was reduced in tumours from rats supplemented with UDCA[16].

In these investigations we also showed that the activating isoform of C/EBPβ was up-regulated in AOM tumours and suppressed by UDCA. C/EBPβ activity is controlled by phosphorylation and required for Ras-dependent transformation in another model of carcinogenesis[39,40]. These results suggest that UDCA inhibits Cox-2 induction by suppressing Ras activity and limiting C/EBPβ expression to reduce Cox-2 transcription in AOM carcinogenesis.

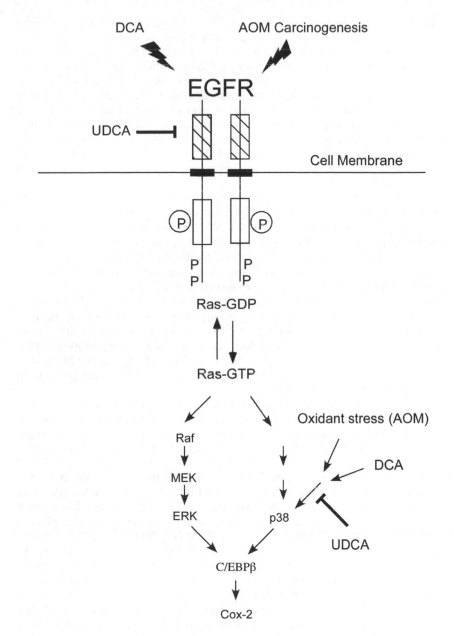

Figure 10 Modulation of EGFR-Ras-kinase signalling pathways by bile acids. AOM induces mutations and oxidant stress that activate EGFR/Ras and p38 signalling and increase C/EBPβ expression to induce Cox-2. DCA enhances these responses, whereas UDCA inhibits EGFR/ Ras and p38 activation and decreases C/EBPβ to limit Cox-2 induction

To dissect the mechanisms by which DCA increases and UDCA inhibits Cox-2 protein expression in colonic carcinogenesis, we examined their effects on Cox-2 promoter activity and mRNA abundance in HCA-7 cells. We found that DCA activated the Cox-2 promoter and induced Cox-2 mRNA and protein in these cells, whereas UDCA suppressed these DCA-induced events. Thus, these bile acids regulate Cox-2 transcription in these cells. These results *in vitro* also parallel our findings *in vivo* that cholic acid increased Cox-2, whereas UDCA suppressed Cox-2 expression in AOM-induced colonic tumours. In addition to transcription, Cox-2 mRNA stability is highly regulated by p38 signalling, and by prostaglandin E2, a Cox-2 product[41]. The role of mRNA stabilization in bile acid effects on Cox-2 expression will require further study[42].

Several signalling pathways, including EGFR/Ras/ERK and p38, regulate Cox-2 expression in HCA-7 cells[27,35]. In our studies we found DCA activated EGFR, Ras and p38. Furthermore, SB 203580 abolished Cox-2 induction at inhibitor concentrations that selectively blocked p38 activity. Our results, taken together with other studies[27,36,43], are consistent with DCA induction of Cox-2 expression via p38- and to a lesser extent ERK-dependent pathway. Consistent with these findings, recent studies have shown that p38 was necessary for Cox-2 induction in premalignant mammary epithelial cells[43]. Based on the ability of DCA to activate the Cox-2 promoter and increase Cox-2 mRNA, this tumour promoting bile acid appears to induce Cox-2 protein expression by increasing gene transcription. We also demonstrated that DCA up-regulates C/EBPβ expression in these cells. We suggest, therefore, that C/EBPβ plays a key role in Cox-2 promoter activation by this bile acid in these cells, and perhaps in colonic malignant transformation.

In contrast to DCA, UDCA inhibited EGFR, Ras and p38 activation *in vitro* and *in vivo*. These effects of UDCA are predicted to inhibit Cox-2 increases, in agreement with our findings. Potential mechanisms by which UDCA might suppress Ras activation in HCA-7 cells include inhibition of up-stream activators such as EGFR. Since UDCA blocked EGFR signalling in normal mouse colon, it is possible that UDCA also inhibits AOM-induced EGFR signalling[25]. Bile acid effects on EGFR signalling in the colon are thought to be detergent-related since no colonic bile acid transporters have been identified[44,45]. DCA is known to deplete cholesterol from the plasma membrane, whereas UDCA antagonizes this effect[46,47]. Furthermore, cholesterol depletion can activate EGFR and Ras, which are known to partition into cholesterol-rich lipid rafts in the plasma membrane[48–50]. AOM and DCA also induce oxidant stress that can activate EGFR and p38[29,51], whereas UDCA induces antioxidant effects[52]. The contrasting effects of these bile acids on lipid raft cholesterol content and oxidant stress probably contribute to their differential effects on EGFR/Ras signalling and Cox-2 induction and their opposing effects on tumorigenesis (Figure 10).

In summary, we have shown in the AOM model that tumour-promoting cholic acid enhanced Ras and p38 activation and induced Cox-2, whereas UDCA inhibited these activations prior to ACF formation. We also found that cholic acid increased Cox-2 expression in AOM tumours, whereas UDCA inhibited this induction. We speculate these effects reflect the ability of UDCA to inhibit EGFR signalling induced by tumorigenesis. In studies *in vitro* we demonstrated that DCA activated EGFR/Ras signalling and induced Cox-2 by a p38 and perhaps C/EBPβ-dependent pathway in HCA-7 cells. In contrast, UDCA decreased Ras activity and inhibited DCA-induced p38 activation and Cox-2 up-regulation in these cells. These opposing signals induced by bile acids probably contribute to their differential effects on colonic carcinogenesis. Further studies to elucidate bile acid-induced pathways regulating Cox-2 expression will identify new or novel targets for chemoprevention.

Acknowledgements

These studies were funded in part by the following grants: P30DK42086 (Digestive Diseases Research Core Center) CA036745 (M.B.), CA097540 (S. K.) and by the Samuel Freedman Research Laboratories for Gastrointestinal Cancer Research. The authors gratefully acknowledge the critical reading of Dr Loren Joseph and Dr Yan-Chun Li.

References

1. Potter JD, Slattery ML, Bostick RM, Gapstur SM. Colon cancer: a review of the epidemiology. Epidemiol Rev. 1993;15:499–545.
2. Lipkin M, Reddy B, Newmark H, Lamprecht SA. Dietary factors in human colorectal cancer. Annu Rev Nutr. 1999;19:545–86.
3. Reddy BS. Dietary fat and colon cancer: animal model studies. Lipids. 1992;27:807–13.
4. Reddy BS, Wynder EL. Metabolic epidemiology of colon cancer. Fecal bile acids and neutral sterols in colon cancer patients and patients with adenomatous polyps. Cancer. 1977;39:2533–9.
5. Weisburger JH, Reddy BS, Barnes WS, Wynder EL. Bile acids, but not neutral sterols, are tumor promoters in the colon in man and in rodents. Environ Health Perspect. 1983;50: 101–7.
6. Nagengast FM, Grubben MJ, van Munster IP. Role of bile acids in colorectal carcinogenesis. Eur J Cancer. 1995;31A:1067–70.
7. Bayerdörffer E, Mannes GA, Ochsenkuhn T et al. Unconjugated secondary bile acids in the serum of patients with colorectal adenomas. Gut. 1995;36:268–73.
8. Earnest DL, Holubec H, Wali RK et al. Chemoprevention of azoxymethane-induced colonic carcinogenesis by supplemental dietary ursodeoxycholic acid. Cancer Res. 1994; 54:5071–4.
9. Baijal PK, Fitzpatrick DW, Bird RP. Comparative effects of secondary bile acids, deoxycholic and lithocholic acids, on aberrant crypt foci growth in the postinitiation phases of colon carcinogenesis. Nutr Cancer. 1998;31:81–9.
10. Sutherland LA, Bird RP. The effect of chenodeoxycholic acid on the development of aberrant crypt foci in the rat colon. Cancer Lett. 1994;76:101–7.
11. Debruyne PR, Bruyneel EA, Li X et al. The role of bile acids in carcinogenesis. Mutat Res. 2001;480–481:359–69.
12. Narahara H, Tatsuta M, Iishi H et al. K-ras point mutation is associated with enhancement by deoxycholic acid of colon carcinogenesis induced by azoxymethane, but not with its attenuation by all-*trans*-retinoic acid. Int J Cancer. 2000;88:157–61.
13. Wali RK, Stoiber D, Nguyen L et al. Ursodeoxycholic acid inhibits the initiation and postinitiation phases of azoxymethane-induced colonic tumor development. Cancer Epidemiol Biomarkers Prev. 2002;11:1316–21.
14. Beuers U, Boyer JL, Paumgartner G. Ursodeoxycholic acid in cholestasis: potential mechanisms of action and therapeutic applications. Hepatology. 1998;28:1449–53.
15. Khare S, Cerda S, Wali RK et al. Ursodeoxycholic acid inhibits ras mutations, wild-type ras activation, and cyclooxygenase-2 expression in colon cancer. Cancer Res. 2003;63:3517–23.

16. Wali R, Khare S, Tretiakova M et al. Ursodeoxycholic acid and F6-D3 inhibit aberrant crypt proliferation in the rat AOM model of colon cancer: roles of cyclin D1 and E-cadherin. Cancer Epidemiol Biomarkers Prev. 2002;11:1653–62.
17. Eberhart CE, Coffey RJ, Radhika A et al. Up-regulation of cyclooxygenase 2 gene expression in human colorectal adenomas and adenocarcinomas. Gastroenterology. 1994; 107:1183–8.
18. DuBois RN, Radhika A, Reddy BS, Entingh AJ. Increased cyclooxygenase-2 levels in carcinogen-induced rat colonic tumors. Gastroenterology. 1996;110:1259–62.
19. Bissonnette M, Khare S, von Lintig FC et al. Mutational and nonmutational activation of p21ras in rat colonic azoxymethane-induced tumors: effects on mitogen-activated protein kinase, cyclooxygenase-2, and cyclin D1. Cancer Res. 2000;60:4602–9.
20. Wang D, Mann JR, DuBois RN. The role of prostaglandins and other eicosanoids in the gastrointestinal tract. Gastroenterology. 2005;128:1445–61.
21. Reddy BS, Hirose Y, Lubet R et al. Chemoprevention of colon cancer by specific cyclooxygenase-2 inhibitor, celecoxib, administered during different stages of carcinogenesis. Cancer Res. 2000;60:293–7.
22. Bird RP, Good CK. The significance of aberrant crypt foci in understanding the pathogenesis of colon cancer. Toxicol Lett. 2000;112–13:395–402.
23. Takayama T, Katsuki S, Takahashi Y et al. Aberrant crypt foci of the colon as precursors of adenoma and cancer. N Engl J Med. 1998;339:1277–84.
24. Baijal PK, Clow EP, Fitzpatrick DW, Bird RP. Tumor-enhancing effects of cholic acid are exerted on the early stages of colon carcinogenesis via induction of aberrant crypt foci with an enhanced growth phenotype. Can J Physiol Pharmacol. 1998;76:1095–102.
25. Im E, Martinez JD. Ursodeoxycholic acid (UDCA) can inhibit deoxycholic acid (DCA)-induced apoptosis via modulation of EGFR/Raf-1/ERK signaling in human colon cancer cells. J Nutr. 2004;134:483–6.
26. Little N, Mustafi R, Cerda S et al. EGFR antagonist Iressa inhibits ERK activation, colonic crypt cell proliferation and ACF growth in mouse azoxymethane model of colon cancer. Gastroenterology. 2005;128:A-175.
27. Shao J, Sheng H, Inoue H, Morrow JD, DuBois RN. Regulation of constitutive cyclooxygenase-2 expression in colon carcinoma cells. J Biol Chem. 2000;275:33951–6.
28. Pearson G, Robinson F, Beers Gibson T et al. Mitogen-activated protein (MAP) kinase pathways: regulation and physiological functions. Endocrinol Rev. 2001;22:153–83.
29. Wilhelm D, Bender K, Knebel A, Angel P. The level of intracellular glutathione is a key regulator for the induction of stress-activated signal transduction pathways including Jun N-terminal protein kinases and p38 kinase by alkylating agents. Mol Cell Biol. 1997;17: 4792–800.
30. Poli V. The role of C/EBP isoforms in the control of inflammatory and native immunity functions. J Biol Chem. 1998;273:29279–82.
31. Rask K, Thorn M, Ponten F et al. Increased expression of the transcription factors CCAAT-enhancer binding protein-beta (C/EBbeta) and C/EBzeta (CHOP) correlate with invasiveness of human colorectal cancer. Int J Cancer. 2000;86:337–43.
32 Bamba H, Ota S, Kato A et al. High expression of cyclooxygenase-2 in macrophages of human colonic adenoma. Int J Cancer. 1999;83:470–5.
33. Caivano M, Gorgoni B, Cohen P, Poli V. The induction of cyclooxygenase-2 mRNA in macrophages is biphasic and requires both CCAAT enhancer-binding protein beta (C/EBP beta) and C/EBP delta transcription factors. J Biol Chem. 2001;276:48693–701.
34. Jagadeeswaran S, Dougherty U, Little N et al. EGFR antagonist Gefitinib inhibits ErbB signaling and tumor development in the rat azoxymethane model of colon cancer. Gastroenterology. 2006;130 (In press).
35. Coffey RJ, Hawkey CJ, Damstrup L et al. Epidermal growth factor receptor activation induces nuclear targeting of cyclooxygenase-2, basolateral release of prostaglandins, and mitogenesis in polarizing colon cancer cells. Proc Natl Acad Sci USA. 1997;94:657–62.
36. Lasa M, Mahtani KR, Finch A et al. Regulation of cyclooxygenase 2 mRNA stability by the mitogen-activated protein kinase p38 signaling cascade. Mol Cell Biol. 2000;20:4265–74.
37. Lee JC, Laydon JT, McDonnell PC et al. A protein kinase involved in the regulation of inflammatory cytokine biosynthesis. Nature. 1994;372:739–46.

38. Tsujii M, DuBois RN. Alterations in cellular adhesion and apoptosis in epithelial cells overexpressing prostaglandin endoperoxide synthase 2. Cell. 1995;83:493–501.
39. Nakajima T, Kinoshita S, Sasagawa T et al. Phosphorylation at threonine-235 by a *ras*-dependent mitogen-activated protein kinase cascade is essential for transcription factor NF-IL6. Proc Natl Acad Sci USA. 1993;90:2207–11.
40. Zhu S, Yoon K, Sterneck E, Johnson PF, Smart RC. CCAAT/enhancer binding protein-beta is a mediator of keratinocyte survival and skin tumorigenesis involving oncogenic Ras signaling. Proc Natl Acad Sci USA. 2002;99:207–12.
41. Faour WH, He Y, He QW et al. Prostaglandin E(2) regulates the level and stability of cyclooxygenase-2 mRNA through activation of p38 mitogen-activated protein kinase in interleukin-1 beta-treated human synovial fibroblasts. J Biol Chem. 2001;276:31720–31.
42. Dixon DA, Tolley ND, King PH et al. Altered expression of the mRNA stability factor HuR promotes cyclooxygenase-2 expression in colon cancer cells. J Clin Invest. 2001;108: 1657–65.
43. Gauthier ML, Pickering CR, Miller CJ et al. p38 regulates cyclooxygenase-2 in human mammary epithelial cells and is activated in premalignant tissue. Cancer Res. 2005;65: 1792–9.
44. Sugimoto Y, Saito H, Tabeta R et al. Binding of bile acids with rat colon and resultant perturbation of membrane organization as studied by uptake measurement and ^{31}P nuclear magnetic resonance spectroscopy. Gann. 1984;75:798–808.
45. Powell AA, LaRue JM, Batta AK, Martinez JD. Bile acid hydrophobicity is correlated with induction of apoptosis and/or growth arrest in HCT116 cells. Biochem J. 2001;356:481–6.
46. Heuman DM, Bajaj R. Ursodeoxycholate conjugates protect against disruptions of cholesterol-rich membranes by bile salts. Gastroenterology. 1994;106:1333–41.
47. Guldutuna S, Deisinger B, Weiss A et al. Ursodeoxycholate stabilizes phospholipid-rich membranes and mimics the effect of cholesterol: investigations on large unilamellar vesicles. Biochim Biophys Acta. 1997;1326:265–74.
48. Puri C, Tosoni D, Comai R et al. Relationships between EGFR signaling-competent and endocytosis-competent membrane microdomains. Mol Biol Cell. 2005;16:2704–18.
49. Mineo C, James GL, Smart EJ, Anderson RG. Localization of epidermal growth factor-stimulated Ras/Raf-1 interaction to caveolae membrane. J Biol Chem. 1996;271:11930–5.
50. Chen X, Resh MD. Cholesterol depletion from the plasma membrane triggers ligand-independent activation of the epidermal growth factor receptor. J Biol Chem. 2002;277:49631–7.
51. Qiao L, Studer E, Leach K et al. Deoxycholic acid (dca) causes ligand-independent activation of epidermal growth factor receptor (egfr) and fas receptor in primary hepatocytes: inhibition of EGFR/mitogen-activated protein kinase- signaling module enhances dca-induced apoptosis. Mol Biol Cell. 2001;12:2629–45.
52. Mitsuyoshi H, Nakashima T, Sumida Y et al. Ursodeoxycholic acid protects hepatocytes against oxidative injury via induction of antioxidants. Biochem Biophys Res Commun. 1999;263:537–42.

Section VI
Colorectal cancer: predictive markers – gene profiling

Chair: S. HAHN and M. VON KNEBEL DOEBERITZ

14
State-of-the-Art Lecture: A gene expression signature to predict recurrence of Dukes' B colon cancer

Y. WANG, T. JATKOE, Y. ZHANG, M. G. MUTCH, D. TALANTOV,
J. JIANG, H. L. McLEOD and D. ATKINS

INTRODUCTION

Like any solid tumour, colon cancer is staged pathologically on the basis of the extent of primary organ involvement and the metastatic spread to lymph nodes or distant organs[1-2]. As 25–30% of the Dukes' B patients would develop tumour relapse, the prognosis signature would provide a powerful tool to select patients at high risk, and ensure that they receive adjuvant treatment. Furthermore, this ability to identify patients who need intensive clinical intervention could lead to an improvement in cancer survival because the benefit of postsurgical chemotherapy in Dukes' B patients has been harder to determine[3-10]. There is clearly a need to identify prognostic factors, in addition to nodal involvement, to guide identification of Dukes' B patients who are likely to relapse. This information would allow more informed planning for patients who are more likely to require and possibly benefit from adjuvant therapy.

DNA microarray-based gene expression profiling technology provides a strategy to search systematically in a combinatorial manner for molecular markers of cancer classification and outcome prediction. The application of genomics to diagnosis and management of cancer is gaining momentum as discovery and initial validation studies are completed[11-16]. The studies suggest that the simultaneous analysis of a large number of genes may offer a powerful and complementary approach to clinical or pathological examination. We reported the results of a highly complex gene expression analysis of 74 Dukes' B colon cancer patients; the result of this analysis has been recently published[17].

PATIENTS AND METHODS

In our study we used frozen tumour specimens from 74 coded Dukes' B colon cancer patients obtained from the Siteman Cancer Center, Washington University School of Medicine (St Louis, MO) and Clinomics (Pittsfield, MA) according to an Institutional Review Board-approved protocol. Archived primary tumour and adjacent non-neoplastic colon tissue were collected at the time of surgery. The histopathology of each specimen was reviewed to confirm diagnosis and uniform involvement with tumour. Regions chosen for analysis contained no normal or benign colon epithelium. Follow-up information was collected from the Division of Colorectal Surgery Patient Database at Washington University and Clinomics. Post-surgery patient surveillance was carried out according to general practice for colon cancer patients including physical examination, blood counts, liver function tests, serum carcinoembryonic antigen (CEA), and colonoscopy for all patients. Selected patients had abdominal computed tomography (CT) scan and chest X-ray. Time to recurrence or disease-free time was defined as the time period from the date of surgery to confirmed tumour relapse date for relapsed patients, and from the date of surgery to the date of last follow-up for disease-free patients.

Total RNA was extracted from each frozen tumour specimen and biotinylated cRNA targets were prepared by using published methods[18]. Targets were hybridized to Affymetrix oligonucleotide microarray U133a GeneChip containing a total of 22 000 probe sets (Santa Clara, CA). For subsequent analysis each probe set was considered as a separate gene. Expression values for each gene were calculated by using Affymetrix GeneChip analysis software MAS 5.0. Gene expression data were first subjected to a filter that excluded genes called 'absent' in all the samples. Of the 22 000 genes considered, 17 616 passed this filter and were used for hierarchical clustering. Prior to the clustering, each gene was divided by its median expression level in patients. This standardization step helped minimize the effect of the magnitude of expression of genes and group together genes with similar patterns of expression in the clustering analysis. Average linkage hierarchical clustering on both the genes and the samples and QT clustering on the genes were performed using GeneSpring 6.0 (San Jose, CA). T-test with Bonferroni corrections was used to identify genes that have different expression levels between two patient subgroups implicated by the clustering result. The Bonferroni corrected p-value of 0.01 was chosen as the threshold for gene selection. The gene with the smallest p value was selected as the indicator to assign patients into the subgroups. Patients in each cluster were further examined with the outcome information.

In order to identify gene markers that can best discriminate the relapse and the disease-free patients, we used the supervised class prediction approaches to select markers from the 17 616 informative genes. The patients were first placed into one of the two subgroups based on the result of the clustering analysis. Each patient subgroup was then analysed separately in order to select markers. The patients in a subgroup were divided into a training set and a testing set with approximately equal numbers of patients. The training set was used to select gene markers. The markers selected from each subgroup were combined to form a single signature to predict tumour recurrence for all patients as a whole. This signature was used in the combined testing set for independent validation. For gene selection, a univariate Cox proportional hazards regression was used to identify genes whose expression levels were correlated to patient disease-free time. A p-value less than 0.02 in the estimated regression coefficients was used as the selection criterion. Secondly, t-test was used to select genes that gave the best classification between the relapse and the disease-free patients ($p < 0.01$). To reduce the chance of distorting the p value caused by outlier patients, resampling 100 times on patients was performed on t-test to search for genes that have a greater than 80% confidence level. In brief, for each resampling, 80% patients in the training set were randomly sampled and a t-test was performed for each gene. After 100 iterations, only genes that gave significant p-values (corrected $p < 0.01$) in more than 80 resamplings were kept for subsequent analysis. Genes found by both Cox model and t-test were selected to build a signature for predicting outcome. The Relapse Hazard Score was used to determine each patient's risk of recurrence. This score was defined as the linear combination of weighted expression with the standardized Cox regression coefficient as the weight. The cutoff for classification was determined using the ROC curve of the training set. The gene signature and the cutoff were validated in the testing set. Kaplan–Meier survival plots and log-rank tests were used to assess the differences in time to recurrence of the predicted high- and low-risk groups. All statistical analyses were performed using S-Plus 6 software (Insightful, VA).

RESULTS AND DISCUSSION

We summarized clinical and pathological features of the patients and their tumours are shown in Table 1. All information on age, gender, tumour size node metastasis (TNM) stage, grade, tumour size and tumour location are included. Seventy-three of the 74 patients had data on the number of lymph nodes that were examined, and 72 of the 74 patients had estimated tumour size information. The patient and tumour characteristics did not differ significantly between the relapse and non-relapse patients. None of the patients received preoperative or postoperative treatment. A minimum of 3 years of follow-up data was available for all the patients in the study.

Unsupervised hierarchical clustering analysis allowed us to cluster the 74 patients on the basis of the similarities of their expression profiles measured over 17 000 informative genes. Distinct patterns of genes were found in the clustering result. Examination of this result led us to identify two patient subgroups that have over 600 differentially expressed genes between them ($p < 0.00001$). Cadherin 17 represented the top gene in the list and thus was selected as the indicator for patient subgroups. The larger subgroup, S1, and the smaller subgroup, S2, contained 54 and 20 patients, respectively. Interestingly, in the larger subgroup of 54 patients only 18 (33%) developed tumour relapse within 3 years, whereas in the smaller subgroup 13 of the 20 patients (65%) had progressive disease (chi square, p-value 0.028). Although the outcome of this subgroup is poor, it is not clear whether this is due to an

Table 1 Patient and tumour characteristics

Factor	Sample distribution	
	Number	%
Age (years)	59 years	
Sex		
Male	33	(45)
Female	41	(55)
T Stage		
T2	17	(23)
T3	55	(74)
T4	2	(3)
Grade		
Good	3	(4)
Moderate	60	(81)
Poor	11	(15)
Metastasis < 3 years		
Yes	31	(42)
No	43	(58)
Censored	0	

incorrect classification by pathological examination for the studied samples or whether it represents a typical make-up of the Dukes' B tumours. We are currently analysing independent sample groups that have similar follow-up data to define this subgroup more precisely.

In order to identify gene markers that can discriminate the relapse and disease-free patients, we divided all 74 patients into a training set and a testing set with approximately equal numbers of patients. The training set was used to select gene markers and to build a prognostic signature. The testing set was used for independent validation. Each patient subgroup was separately analysed in order to select markers. Seven genes were selected from the training set of subgroup 1 and 15 genes were selected from the training set of subgroup 2. Taking together the selected genes and cadherin 17, a Cox model to predict patient recurrence was built to predict the Dukes' B patients as a whole. The functional annotation for these genes provides an insight into the underlying biological mechanism leading to rapid metastases. Both tumour cell- and immune cell-expressed genes have been implicated as prognostic factors for predicting tumour recurrence.

We next produced the ROC curves for each of them using the 36 independent patients in the testing set. The parameter that was used to assess the performance of a predictor was the area under the curve (AUC). The 23-gene predictor generated an AUC of 0.74. To summarize the validation result of the 23-gene prognostic signature the 36 patients in the testing set included 27

Table 2 Univariate and multivariate analysis for distant recurrence

	Univariate analysis			Multivariate analysis[a]		
	HR[b]	(95% CI)	p-Value	HR	(95% CI)	p-Value
Age	0.99	(0.95–1.04)	0.8934	0.99	(0.95–1.04)	0.7115
Sex[c]	0.66	(0.26–1.71)	0.3931	0.72	(0.26–2.01)	0.5330
T stage	1.38	(0.62–3.09)	0.4319	2.46	(0.83–7.29)	0.1055
Grade[d]	1.03	(0.24–4.51)	0.9698	0.99	(0.19–5.28)	0.9921
Tumour size[e]	1.09	(0.43–2.76)	0.8634	0.82	(0.29–2.33)	0.7092
23-gene signature	4.06	(1.42–11.6)	0.0091	5.38	(1.75–16.5)	0.0033

[a]The multivariate model includes 35 patients, due to missing values in one patient.

[b]Hazard ratio.

[c]Sex: male vs female.

[d]Grade: moderate and well vs poor.

[e]Tumour size: ⩾5 mm vs <5 mm.

153

patients from subgroup 1 and nine patients from subgroup 2. Furthermore, it consisted of 18 patients who developed tumour relapses within 3 years and 18 patients who remained disease-free for more than 3 years. The prediction resulted in 13 correct relapse classifications and 15 correct disease-free classifications. The overall performance accuracy is 78% (28 of 36) with a sensitivity of 72% (13 of 18) and a specificity of 83% (15 of 18). This performance would indicate that the Dukes' B patients who have a relapse hazard score above the threshold of the prognostic signature have a 13-fold odds ratio (95% CI 2.6–65; $p = 0.003$) to develop tumour relapse within 3 years compared with those who have a relapse hazard score below the threshold of the prognostic signature. In the univariate and multivariate Cox proportional hazards regression, the estimated hazard ratios for tumour recurrence is 4.06 and 5.36 respectively, indicating that the 23-gene set represents a prognostic signature that is inversely associated with a higher risk of tumour recurrence (Table 2).

We report the successful prediction of outcome in Dukes' B colon cancer patients using a 23-gene signature derived from microarray gene expression data and classification methods. As an initial example our selection of multivariate patterns in gene expression data from the primary tumours and examination of the value of such patterns in prediction of independent testing samples resulted in a predictive accuracy of 78% in the independent samples. This represented an odds ratio of 13 (95% CI between 2.6 and 65, $p = 0.003$) that is much higher than the characterized prognostic factors in colon cancer, such as lymph node status. As expected, genes implicated in recurrence prediction do not show a striking functional clustering but include multiple features previously associated with colon cancer progression. The genes in the signature include those that regulate cell proliferation, cell signalling and immune responses. Our study strongly indicates that colon cancer prognosis can be derived from the gene expression profile of the primary tumour. The results also demonstrate the potential of DNA microarray-based recognition of gene expression patterns for the prediction of patient outcome in colon cancer. This is likely to have an impact on current clinical practice for the eligibility of adjuvant chemotherapy on treatment of Dukes' B colon cancer patients.

References

1. Liefers GJ, Cleton-Jansen AM, van de Velde CJ et al. Micrometastases and survival in stage II colorectal cancer. N Engl J Med. 1998;339:223–8.
2. Markowitz SD, Dawson DM, Willis J et al. Focus on colon cancer. Cancer Cell. 2002;1: 233–6.
3. Caplin S, Cerottini JP, Bosman FT et al. For patients with Dukes' B (TNM Stage II) colorectal carcinoma, examination of six or fewer lymph nodes is related to poor prognosis. Cancer. 1998;83:666–72.
4. Compton CC, Fielding LP, Burgart LJ et al. Prognostic factors in colorectal cancer. College of American Pathologists Consensus Statement 1999. Arch Pathol Lab Med. 2000;124:979–94
5. Wolmark N, Rockette H, Mamounas E et al. Clinical trial to assess the relative efficacy of fluorouracil and leucovorin, fluorouracil and levamisole, and fluorouracil, leucovorin, and levamisole in patients with Dukes' B and C carcinoma of the colon: results from National Surgical Adjuvant Breast and Bowel Project C-04. J Clin Oncol. 1999;17:3553–9.

6. International multicenter pooled analysis of B2 colon cancer trials (IMPACT B2) investigators: efficacy of adjuvant fluorouracil and folinic acid in B2 colon cancr. J Clin Oncol. 1999;17:1356–63.

7. Mamounas E, Wieand S, Wolmark N et al. Comparative efficacy of adjuvant chemotherapy in patients with Dukes' B versus Dukes' C colon cancer: results from four National Surgical Adjuvant Breast and Bowel Project adjuvant studies (C-01, C-02, C-03, and C-04). J Clin Oncol. 1999;17:1349–55.

8. McLeod HL, Murray GI. Tumor markers of prognosis in colorectal cancer. Br J Cancer. 1999;79:191–203.

9. Allen WL, Johnston PG. Have we made progress in pharmacogenomics? The implementation of molecular markers in colon cancer. Pharmacogenomics. 2005;6:603–14.

10. Allen WL, Johnston PG. Role of genomic markers in colorectal cancer treatment. J Clin Oncol. 2005;23:4545–52.

11. Van't Veer LJ, Dai H, van de Vijver MJ et al. Gene expression profiling predicts clinical outcome of breast cancer. Nature. 2002;415:530–6.

12. Beer DG, Kardia SLR, Huang C et al. Gene expression profiles predict survival of patients with lung adenocarcinoma. Nature Med. 2002;8:816–24.

13. Shipp MA, Ross KN, Tamayo P et al. Diffuse large B-cell lymphoma outcome prediction by gene-expression profiling and supervised machine learning. Nature Med. 2002;8:68–74.

14. Ransohoff DF. Bias as a threat to the validity of cancer molecular-marker research. Nat Rev Cancer. 2005;5:142–9.

15. Simon R, Radmacher MD, Dobbin K et al. Pitfalls in the use of DNA microarray data for diagnostic and prognostic classification. J Natl Cancer Inst. 2003;95:14–18.

16. Rosenwald A, Wright G, Chan WC et al. The use of molecular profiling to predict survival after chemotherapy for diffuse larger B-cell lymphoma. N Engl J Med. 2002;346:1937–47.

17. Wang Y, Jatkoe, T, Zhang, Y et al. Gene expression profiles and molecular markers to predict recurrence of Dukes' B colon cancer. J Clin Oncol. 2004;22:1564–71.

18. Lipshutz RJ, Fodor SP, Gingeras TR et al. High density synthetic oligonucleotide arrays. Nature Genet. 1999;21:20–4.

15
Chromosomal deletions as predictors for recurrence of early stage colorectal cancer

W. ZHOU

EARLY STAGE COLORECTAL TUMOUR AND ITS RECURRENCE

The incidence of colorectal cancer (CRC) ranks third in frequency in the world with an estimated 1 million new cases and half a million deaths[1]. Disease progression and treatment options are usually determined based on tumour staging, and the international standard of CRC staging in all disciplines is the tumour, node, metastasis (TNM) staging system of the American Joint Committee on Cancer (AJCC)[2] and the International Union against Cancer (UICC)[3]. In general, patients with metastatic disease (stage III, involving lymph nodes, and stage IV, involving distant sites) have a poor prognosis and receive adjuvant therapy. Early-stage patients who present without metastases (stage I and II), on the other hand, have much better disease prognosis, and may require only local surgical treatment. Nevertheless, a significant fraction (10–30%) of early-stage patients develop recurrences and die from the disease.

Treatment benefit of adjuvant chemotherapies is controversial in early-stage CRC patients. While an analysis of four separate studies (National Surgical Adjuvant Breast and Bowel Project) compared the benefit of adjuvant treatment in Dukes' B patients with that in Dukes' C patients, and showed similar relative reductions in mortality and disease-free survival in Dukes' B and in Dukes' C patients, the International Multicenter Pooled Analysis of Colon Cancer Trials B2 study, which combined data from patients with Dukes' B colon cancer in five separate trials, failed to show a statistically significant benefit of adjuvant 5-FU/leucovorin compared with surgery alone[4]. A meta-analysis of all adjuvant trials may reliably address this issue, but even if adjuvant chemotherapies do improve long-term survival, and are recommended for all early-stage patients, this still would not negate the fact that these therapies are associated with various side-effects and many early-stage CRC patients will receive unnecessary adjuvant treatment after the removal of a primary tumour. It obviously would be valuable to be able to predict which patients without clinical or pathological evidence of metastatic disease are likely to suffer recurrences. This information would allow more informed planning for the future, and facilitate selection of patients who are most likely to benefit from adjuvant therapies.

MOLECULAR PREDICTOR FOR EARLY-STAGE CRC

In light of the importance of this issue there have been numerous attempts to identify novel molecular markers that can predict CRC disease progression. The most successful markers so far are the ones that can identify microsatellite instability (MIN). Unlike the human genome in normal tissues, which contains 23 pairs of chromosomes and a stable genome, the tumour genome is a dynamic, unstable entity and constantly undergoes changes due to defects in the DNA repair and mitotic checkpoint machineries. These perpetual, gene-altering activities result in either microsatellite instability (MIN) or chromosome instability (CIN)[5,6]. Approximately 13% of sporadic CRC are MIN type tumour and the majority of them are CIN tumours[7]. Extensive evidence indicates that patients with MIN tumours have a significantly better disease prognosis. A recent systematic review of 32 studies indicated the hazards ratio (HR) for overall survival associated with MIN was 0.65 (95% CI 0.59–0.71), and this benefit was maintained restricting analyses to clinical trial patients (HR = 0.69; 95% CI 0.56 0.85) and patients with locally advanced colorectal cancer (HR = 0.67; 95% CI 0.58–0.78)[7]. Since the majority of MIN tumour patients have a better prognosis, existing data suggested that these patients derived no benefit from adjuvant fluorouracil treatment.

The majority of CRC have CIN, and allelic imbalance analysis has been the main focus to date. An initial report in 1994 by Jen et al. indicated that disease prognosis in patients with stage II cancer and chromosome 18q allelic loss is similar to that in patients with stage III cancer, who may benefit from adjuvant therapy. In contrast, patients with stage II disease who do not have chromosome 18q allelic loss in their tumour have a survival rate similar to that of patients with stage I disease and may not require additional therapy[8]. The confirmation of this initial observation has been controversial. A recent systematic analysis of pooled data from 2189 cases from 17 studies showed significantly worse overall survival in patients with chromosome 18q loss, but the authors noted evidence of heterogeneity and publication bias[9].

PROBLEMS ASSOCIATED WITH THE TRADITIONAL ALLELIC IMBALANCE ANALYSIS METHOD

There are many potential reasons for this observed heterogeneity and publication bias. One of them is the use of archived clinical specimens. Retrospective genetic analysis is a powerful tool in studying the associations between genetic alterations and the natural history of disease progression. The identification of fresh or frozen tumour samples with associated demographic or clinical data is still a new endeavour for most hospitals, and many years may pass before the process has matured sufficiently to enable the prospective study of natural history of cancer progression. Until fresh-frozen tissue banking truly arrives, most retrospective analyses must be conducted with fixed archived specimens, such as paraffin-embedded primary tumours. Such specimens, however, have several unique features and require special experimental considerations.

1. Tissue heterogeneity. Primary tumours contain both tumour and normal cells, and the presence of normal cells from stroma, normal epithelial cells, endothelial cells and infiltrating lymphocytes represents one level of heterogeneity. The first experimental challenge is to eliminate experimental errors introduced by normal contaminants.

2. Tumour heterogeneity. There is also genetic heterogeneity within the tumour cell population as the tumour genome is not stable. Consequently, each tumour cell may contain many genetic alterations, most of which are byproducts of genetic instability and will not provide any information regarding prognosis. Hence, the second experimental challenge is to identify genetic alterations that are involved in clonal expansion and are present in the majority of tumour cells, not just in individual tumour cells. This issue becomes important when microdissection techniques are used for the procurement of pure tumour tissues and only a few tumour tissues are recovered for analyses.

3. Tissue integrity. Archived paraffin-embedded samples are the most common clinical specimens for retrospective analyses. However, they are stored at ambient temperature for extended periods, and nucleic acids in these preserved tissues could be degraded to various extents. Hence, the third experimental challenge is to accurately assess specific alterations of tumour cells in compromised tissue specimens.

These unique properties of archived specimens rendered the traditional allelic imbalance method using microsatellite repeats inadequate. The standard assay involves PCR amplification of a specific microsatellite with a pair of adjacent primers in the presence of a radioisotope. Since microsatellite repeats are different in length, the polymorphic alleles can be resolved by polyacrylamide gel electrophoresis (PAGE). Allelic loss is determined by the absence of one allele in the tumour sample compared to the paired normal. This assay was originally designed for family-based linkage analysis with genetically pure cell populations, and it could be used to test loss of heterozygosity (LOH) in cancer cell lines and xenografts (pure cell population). However, several issues complicate its utility in primary tumours.

1. DNA isolated from archived tissues may be contaminated with a small fraction of normal tissue, which contains both alleles. The contaminating allele can be amplified and conceal the true allelic loss in tumour.

2. Microsatellite repeats are different in length, and larger alleles may be more susceptible to DNA degradation in tumour cells undergoing apoptosis or necrosis. A meta-analysis of 88 LOH studies showed that larger alleles were lost significantly more frequently than smaller alleles, indicating an artifactual bias due to preferential DNA degradation of larger alleles[10].

3. Most laboratories use a larger than 50% reduction in allele intensities on an autoradiogram as a criterion for allelic loss. Such a criterion is non-quantitative and somewhat subjective, which is prone to mistakes.

OPTIMIZING ALLELIC IMBALANCE ANALYSIS IN ARCHIVED SPECIMENS USING SINGLE-NUCLEOTIDE POLYMORPHIC MARKERS

To address the common issues associated with allelic imbalance analysis in primary tumours we have recently developed a technique called 'counting alleles'[11], using a digital PCR method[12]. This method is quantitative and is not susceptible to PCR amplification-bias and DNA degradation. Hence, it is more suitable for LOH analysis in archived clinical specimens. Here are the unique features of the 'counting alleles' method

1. Single nucleotide polymorphic (SNP) markers are used instead of microsatellites. SNP are biallelic polymorphic markers that are identical in length (1 bp), thus not susceptible to size-based amplification bias.

2. The detection of different alleles of each SNP locus is carried out with SNP-specific molecular beacons (MB) and does not require the use of radioisotope or gel electrophoresis.

3. Allelic status of a sample is determined quantitatively by directly counting the number of alleles in a sample. Normal tissues and tumours without LOH will have approximately equal numbers for both alleles. Tumour samples with chromosomal loss and normal tissue contaminations will have different numbers for two alleles.

4. The presence or absence of alleles in a sample is determined by a statistical approach, the sequential probability ratio test (SPRT). This test can determine whether a specific tumour specimen contains allelic loss with up to 50% normal tissue contamination.

An initial study using the 'counting allele' technique involved 78 early-stage CRC patients. It revealed a correlation between 18q loss and vascular invasion in node-negative tumours[13]. Subsequent analysis with 198 CRC patients demonstrated that early-stage patients could be stratified into three groups with 0%, 27% and 48% chance of recurrence based on allelic status of 8p and 18q[14]. For patients with allelic imbalance of both 18p and 18, disease prognosis was poor even if the patients had stage I disease. The ability to predict which of these patients might develop a recurrence would obviously be of great benefit for prognostication and treatment planning.

Mechanistically, this observed association between 8p/18q allelic imbalance and disease progression could be due to either the inactivation of critical tumour-suppressor genes on these two chromosomes or the overall level of chromosome alterations accumulated during tumour development, i.e. the more advanced tumours will accumulate more chromosome alteration, and thus be more likely to have allelic imbalance in both chromosomes 8p and 18q. To clarify this issue we have recently completed similar 8p/18q analysis in early-stage prostate and breast cancer[15,16]. 8p/18q allelic loss are not associated with disease progression in these two cancer types, suggesting that the association observed in CRC is due to the inactivation of tumour-suppressor genes that play important roles in the recurrence of early-stage colorectal cancer. The identities of these genes, however, are still unknown.

ALLELIC IMBALANCE ANALYSIS WITH SNP IN THE FUTURE

The current 'counting alleles' method is not a high-throughput method. In addition, reagent cost for each assay is approximately $40, and a robotic system is required for the experiment setup. To circumvent these limitations, 'BEAMing' method was recently developed by Dressman et al.[17]. In brief, DNA primers are coupled to magnetic particles, and single molecule amplifications were carried out in water-in-oil microemulsions where each DNA molecule was amplified with a single magnetic bead to yield thousands of copies of DNA identical in sequence to the original on the bead. Therefore, the final population of beads corresponds to a one-to-one representation of the starting DNA molecules. Variation within the original DNA molecules can then be determined by counting fluorescently labelled particles via flow cytometry. Using this technique, millions of individual DNA molecules can be assessed with standard laboratory equipment, while the reagent cost is reduced by 90%. The BEAMing technique has been successfully reproduced by over a dozen laboratories, and be easily adapted for allelic imbalance analysis.

Many commercial SNP products and services are now available for allelic imbalance analysis[18]. Among these, high-density oligonucleotide arrays from Affymetrix (HuSNP array) offer a high-throughput method for the parallel analysis of thousands of SNP in a single experiment. The feasibility of SNP array-based genome-wide allelic imbalance analysis was first demonstrated with the prototype SNP array containing 600 biallelic markers for the analysis of benign neurofibromatosis type 2 (NF-2) tumours and malignant oesophageal adenocarcinomas[19]. The current HuSNP array consists of the 500 K array, 100 K array, and 10 K arrays, and requires only 120 ng of starting genomic DNA per assay (http://www.affymetrix.com). Early studies using such an array demonstrated that this SNP array can be reliably employed for assessing allelic losses but not for detecting modest increases in chromosome copy numbers in small cell lung carcinoma (SCLC). In addition, this group demonstrated that HuSNP arrays can tolerate up to 10% contamination with normal tissues[20]. Nevertheless, extensive efforts have been devoted to the optimization of this method, and recent studies suggested that this approach may be suitable for archived specimen analysis with improved software[21].

Acknowledgements

This work was supported by the American Cancer Society (RSG CCE-108980 to W.Z.) and the Department of Defense (Idea Development Award PC040315). W.Z. is a Georgia Cancer Coalition distinguished Cancer Scholar.

Reference

1. Parkin DM, Bray F, Ferlay J, Pisani P. Global cancer statistics, 2002. Cancer J Clin. 2005;55:74–108.
2. Greene FL, Page DL, Fleming ID. AJCC Cancer Staging Manual, 6th edn. New York: Springer, 2002.
3. Sobin LH, Wittekind C. TNM: Classification of Malignant Tumours, 6th edn. New York: Wiley-Liss, 2002.
4. Buyse M, Piedbois P. Should Dukes' B patients receive adjuvant therapy? A statistical perspective. Semin Oncol. 2001;28:20–4.
5. Lengauer C, Kinzler KW, Vogelstein B. Genetic instability in colorectal cancers. Nature. 1997;386:623–7.
6. Lengauer C, Kinzler KW, Vogelstein B. Genetic instabilities in human cancers. Nature. 1998;396:643–9.
7. Popat S, Hubner R, Houlston RS. Systematic review of microsatellite instability and colorectal cancer prognosis. J Clin Oncol. 2005;23:609–18.
8. Jen J, Kim H, Piantadosi S et al. Allelic loss of chromosome 18q and prognosis in colorectal cancer. N Engl J Med. 1994;331:213–21.
9. Popat S, Houlston RS. A systematic review and meta-analysis of the relationship between chromosome 18q genotype, DCC status and colorectal cancer prognosis. Eur J Cancer. 2005;41:2060–70.
10. Liu J, Zabarovska VI, Braga E, Alimov A, Klien G, Zabarovsky ER. Loss of heterozygosity in tumor cells requires re-evaluation: the data are biased by the size-dependent differential sensitivity of allele detection. FEBS Lett. 1999;462:121–8.
11. Zhou W, Williams T, Colpaert C, Morikawa A, Zhong D. Digital PCR analysis of allelic status in clinical specimens. In: VV Demidov, NE Broude, editors. DNA Amplification: Current Technologies and Applications Norfolk: Horizon Bioscience, 2004.
12. Vogelstein B, Kinzler KW. Digital PCR. Proc Natl Acad Sci USA. 1999;96:9236–41.
13. Zhou W, Galizia G, Lieto E et al. Counting alleles reveals a connection between chromosome 18q loss and vascular invasion. Nat Biotechnol. 2001;19:78–81.
14. Zhou W, Goodman SN, Galizia G et al. Counting alleles to predict recurrence of early-stage colorectal cancers. Lancet. 2002;359:219–25.
15. Morikawa A, Williams TY, Dirix L et al. Allelic imbalances of chromosome 8p and 18q and their roles in distant relapse of early stage, node-negative breast cancer. Breast Cancer Res. 2005;7:R1051–7.
16. Zhou W, Goodman M, Lyles R et al. Surgical margin and Gleason score as predictors of post-operative recurrence in prostate cancer with or without chromosome 8p allelic imbalance. Prostate. 2004;61:81–91.
17. Dressman D, Yan H, Traverso G, Kinzler KW, Vogelstein B. Transforming single DNA molecules into fluorescent magnetic particles for detection and enumeration of genetic variations. Proc Natl Acad Sci USA. 2003;100:8817–22.
18. Wypgant M. SNP market view: opportunities, technologies, and products. Biotechniques. 2002;(Suppl.)78–80, 82, 84 passim.
19. Mei R, Galipeau PC, Prass C et al. Genome-wide detection of allelic imbalance using human SNPs and high-density DNA arrays. Genome Res. 2000;10:1126–37.
20. Lindblad-Toh K, Tanenbaum DM, Daly MJ et al. Loss-of-heterozygosity analysis of small-cell lung carcinomas using single-nucleotide polymorphism arrays. Nat Biotechnol. 2000; 18:1001–5.
21. Lin M, Wei LJ, Sellers WR, Lieberfarb M, Wong WH, Li C. dChipSNP: significance curve and clustering of SNP-array-based loss-of-heterozygosity data. Bioinformatics. 2004;20: 1233–40.

Section VII
Colorectal cancer:
interdisciplinary treatment

Chair: W. HOHENBERGER and C. LOUVET

16
Resection or local ablation of colorectal cancer metastasis to the liver – pro and con

H.-P. ALLGAIER

The optimal treatment for patients with colorectal cancer (CRC) metastases confined to the liver is surgical resection when adequate margins are feasible. Unfortunately, many patients with CRC liver metastases are not eligible for hepatic resection. Factors that preclude curative surgery include tumour location in close proximity to hilar structures, poor performance status, or inadequate hepatic reserve. Therefore, interest has focused on alternative treatment strategies. Direct thermal ablation treatments using laser, microwaves, or radiofrequency, are frequently used in clinical practice. Furthermore, the majority of patients who undergo resection of CRC liver metastases eventually develops recurrent disease.

Radiofrequency thermal ablation (RFA) was first described in 1990 by Rossi and McGahan. RFA can be applied percutaneously as well as during open or laparoscopic surgery, and probe placement can be guided by ultrasonography (US), computed tomography (CT), or magnetic resonance imaging (MRI). Commercially available RFA probes have a diameter of 14–21G and induce frictional heat within tissue. A cytotoxic effect is observed at 41°C; immediate coagulation necrosis occurs at 90°C. The two main strategies that have been developed to increase the amount of ablated tumour tissue are saline cooled-tip needles and expandable-array systems.

RF ablation of malignant liver lesions can usually be performed under local anaesthesia. After US-guided puncture of the tumour a coagulation necrosis is induced with a temperature of about 90°C. Multiple temperature sensors are located at the tips of the electrode, allowing precise monitoring. Finally, the puncture track is carefully ablated[1].

Studies have shown practical difficulties in assessing the adequacy of ablation. The lack of enhancement after contrast injection indicates necrotic tissue in contrast-enhanced US, CT or MRI. Sometimes a surrounding rim of hypervascular tissue is observed, which can be associated with post-ablation change, but might also contain viable tumour.

Several reports have demonstrated the efficacy and safety of RFA in hepatic CRC metastases. Interpretation of these data is challenging given that many of these reports describe a variety of tumour types and different RFA techniques. Published series have shown local recurrence rates ranging from 8% to 34%. Recurrence rates are a function of the size of the ablated lesion.

Most investigators agree that the rate of local recurrence after ablation of tumours larger than 4 cm is unacceptably high. Other predictors of failure, in a review of 250 ablations for liver tumours, included inadequate RFA technique and vascular invasion. In a review of 1931 patients treated with RFA, 10 treatment-related deaths (0.5%) were reported. Major complications occurred in 137 patients (7%) and the most common complications were impairment of hepatic function, haemorrhage, and infection[2].

The increasing availability of sophisticated techniques for liver imaging, e.g. contrast-enhanced US, should lead to more precise identification of liver lesions. Furthermore, use of stereoscopic three-dimensional localization techniques in radiofrequency-probe technology should lead to more precise ablation, and research on probe technology will continue to develop more effective and safe methods to deliver thermal energy.

In summary, RFA is a safe and effective treatment option to destroy malignant liver tumours. In the majority of patients only a single intervention is necessary. RFA is characterized by low morbidity, mortality and costs. RFA can be applied percutaneously as well as during open or laparoscopic surgery. RFA has a favourable safety profile relative to other ablative methods and its potential synergy with systemic chemotherapy needs to be analysed in large randomized studies.

Technical limitations of RFA exist in tumours located near large vessels by heat generation resulting in an incomplete necrosis ('heat sink effect'). In the majority of patients needle tract ablation should prevent tumour seeding. The local recurrence rate after RFA is relatively high and is a function of the size of the ablated lesion. Further, inadequate RFA technique and vascular invasion predict local recurrence.

In conclusion, patients with liver tumours should undergo multidisciplinary assessment, and RFA should be performed only after consideration of all therapeutic options available. While RFA is an interesting and promising therapy for the treatment of liver metastases, the evidence available to date does not support the use of this technique as a single treatment modality for patients with non-resectable liver metastases. Clear evidence for a survival benefit after treatment with RFA is not yet available.

References

1. Lencioni R, Crocetti L, Cioni D, Della Pina C, Bartolozzi C. Percutaneous radiofrequency ablation of hepatic colorectal metastases: technique, indications, results, and new promises. Invest Radiol. 2004;39:689–97.
2. Siriwardena AK. Radiofrequency ablation of liver tumours: systematic review. Lancet Oncol. 2004;5:550–60.

17
Radiation therapy for rectal cancer: neoadjuvant or adjuvant?

C. RÖDEL

INTRODUCTION

New data have been collected and progress has been made both in surgery and perioperative radio-(chemo)therapy for rectal cancer in recent years. Better knowledge of microscopic lymphatic spread within the mesorectum has led to the use of total mesorectal excision for mid and low rectal cancer. With this 'optimized' surgery, local control rates have been markedly increased and local failure rates above 15–20% are now no longer acceptable. Technical advances in radiotherapy, including tumour- and radiobiologically optimized fractionation, 3-D treatment planning and intensity-modulated radiation therapy will further allow application of more sophisticated treatment volume to reduce irradiation of normal tissue and increase the therapeutic index. Moreover, novel chemotherapeutic and biological agents, e.g. capecitabine, oxaliplatin, irinotecan, cetuximab, and bevacizumab, are currently incorporated in multimodality regimens.

RANDOMIZED TRIALS OF POSTOPERATIVE RADIOTHERAPY, CHEMOTHERAPY OR COMBINED RADIOCHEMOTHERAPY IN LOCALLY ADVANCED RECTAL CANCER

Historically, in rectal cancer, the combination of postoperative radiotherapy and 5-fluorouracil (5-FU)-based chemotherapy has been shown in several randomized trials to reduce local recurrence rates and to improve overall survival compared with (conventional) surgery alone or surgery plus postoperative radiotherapy (Table 1)[1–6]. The NCI Consensus Conference concluded in 1990 that combined radiochemotherapy was the standard adjuvant treatment for patients with tumour node metastasis (TNM) stages II and III rectal cancer[7].

Table 1 Randomized trials of postoperative radiation, chemotherapy, or combined radiochemotherapy for locally advanced rectal cancer (UICC II and III)

Series	Treatment	Local failure (%)	Distant failure (%)	5-Year-survival (%)
GITSG 7175 (Gastrointestinal Tumor Study Group 1985)[1]	Surgery	24	34	45
	Surgery + RT	20 ($p = 0.08$)	30	52 ($p < 0.05$)
	Surgery + 5-FU/MeCCNU	27	27	56
	Surgery + RT-5-FU/ MeCCNU	11	26	59
NCCTG/Mayo 794751 (Krook et al. 1991)[2]	Surgery + RT	25	46 ($p = 0.01$)	48 ($p = 0.025$)
	Surgery + RT + 5-FU/MeCCNU	13.5	29	58
Norway trial (Tveit et al. 1997)[3]	Surgery	30 ($p = 0.01$)	39	50 ($p = 0.05$)
	Surgery + RT + 5-FU	12	33	64
NSABP R-01 (Fisher et al. 1988)[4]	Surgery	25 ($p = 0.06$)	26	43
	Surgery + RT	16	31	41
	Surgery + MOF	21	24	53
NSABP R-02 (Wolmark et al. 2000)[5]	Surgery + CT*	13 ($p = 0.02$)	29	64
	Surgery + RCT	8	31	64
Italy trial (Cafiero et al. 2003)[6]	Surgery + RT	20	38	59
	Surgery + 5-FU/LEV + RT + 5-FU/LEV (RT and CT applied sequentially)	22	27	43

*Male patients received MOF (MeCCNU, Vincristin, 5-FU) or 5-FU/LV; female patients only 5-FU/LV.

CT, chemotherapy; 5-FU, 5-fluorouracil; LEV, levamisol; LV, leucovorin; MeCCNU, 1-(2-chloroethyl)-3-(4-methylcyclohexyl)-1-nitrosourea; RCT, radiochemotherapy; RT, radiotherapy.

RANDOMIZED TRIALS TO OPTIMIZE THE ADMINISTRATION OF 5-FU-BASED POSTOPERATIVE RADIOCHEMOTHERAPY

Further trials by the GITSG (7180) and NCCTG (864751) investigated the need for methyl CCNU in the chemotherapy regimen and found that it added no benefit to the 5-FU regimen (Table 2)[8,9]. Thus, this compound is no longer used for adjuvant radiochemotherapy in rectal cancer. NCCTG (864751) also tested the best method of administering 5-FU during radiotherapy: bolus 5-FU (500 mg/m^2 for 3 days during weeks 1 and 5 of radiation therapy) was compared with protracted infusion (225 mg/m^2 during the whole course of radiotherapy): a 10% disease-free and overall survival advantage was achieved with 5-FU continuous infusion during radiotherapy.

The INT 0144 trail tested the question whether additional continuous-infusion 5-FU instead of bolus 5-FU before and after radiochemotherapy (or modulation of 5-FU through addition of leucovorin and levamisol) may further increase tumour control. Data were reported at ASCO 2003 and showed no difference in 3-year survival[10]. Results of a four-arm intergroup trial, INT 0114, also showed no significant differences in local control and survival among patients receiving either bolus 5-FU, bolus 5-FU + folinic acid, bolus 5-FU + levamisol, or bolus 5-FU + folinic acid + levamisol[11]. However, gastrointestinal toxicity was higher in folinic acid-containing regimens. The largest German adjuvant rectal cancer trial (FOGT 2) compared 5-FU + levamisol to 5-FU + levamisol + folinic acid and 5-FU + levamisol + interferon alpha as systemic treatment added to 45–50.4 Gy of radiotherapy. Toxicity was highest in the interferon-containing arm, that was closed prematurely. Long-term results showed no difference in failure rates and survival between the other groups[12].

Given all these results, the standard design of postoperative radiochemotherapy is to deliver six cycles of 5-FU chemotherapy with concurrent radiation therapy during cycles 3 and 4. During radiotherapy continuous-infusion 5-FU regimens (e.g. 225 mg/m^2 per day during the whole course of radiation, or 1000 mg/m^2 per day as 120 h continuous infusion during weeks 1 and 5 of radiation, as in the German CAO/ARO/AIO-95-study, see below) are recommended. A recent randomized Korean trial (Table 2) suggests that radiation should start with cycle 1 rather than 3, which supports the radiobiological paradigm that subclinical disease in the pelvis is best controlled if radiochemotherapy is applied as soon as possible after surgical resection to account for any regrowth of residual tumour cells[13].

RANDOMIZED TRIALS TO OPTIMIZE THE SEQUENCE OF COMBINED MODALITY TREATMENT: THE CONCEPT OF PREOPERATIVE RADIOCHEMOTHERAPY

The interest in preoperative radiochemotherapy for resectable tumours of the rectum is based not only on the success of the combined-modality approach in the postoperative setting, but also on many radio-biological and tumour-biological advantages of the preoperative approach. Among those are

Table 2 Randomized trials of postoperative combined radiochemotherapy in locally advanced rectal cancer

Series	Treatment	DFS	OS
GITSG 7180 (GITSG 1992)[8]	RCT bolus 5-FU + bolus 5-FU (6 cycles, escalating 5-FU) RCT bolus 5-FU + bolus 5-FU/MeCCNU (12 months treatment)	68% (3 years) 54% (3 years) $p = 0.20$	75% (3 years) 66% (3 years) $p = 0.58$
NCCTG 864751 (O'Connell et al. 1994)[9]	2 cycles of bolus 5-FU ($\pm$MeCCNU) + RCT bolus 5-FU + 2 cycles of bolus 5-FU ($\pm$MeCCNU) 2 cycles of bolus 5-FU ($\pm$MeCCNU) + RCT PVI 5-FU + 2 cycles of bolus 5-FU ($\pm$MeCCNU)	53% (4 years) 63% (4 years) $p = 0.01$	60% (4 years) 70% (4 years) $p = 0.005$
Hellenic Trial (Fountzilas et al. 1999)[22]	1 cycle 5 FU/LV + RCT bolus 5-FU + 3 cycles 5-FU/LV RCT bolus 5-FU	70 % (3 years) 68% (3 years) $p = 0.53$	77% (3 years) 73% (3 years) $p = 0.75$
INT 0114 (Tepper et al. 2002)[11]	2 cycles bolus 5-FU + RCT bolus 5-FU + 2 cycles bolus 5-FU 2 cycles bolus 5-FU/LV + RCT bolus 5-FU/LV + 2 cycles bolus 5-FU/LV 2 cycles bolus 5-FU/LEV + RCT bolus 5-FU/LV + 2 cycles bolus 5-FU/LEV 2 cycles bolus 5-FU/LV/LEV + RCT bolus 5-FU/LV/LEV + 2 cycles bolus 5-FU/LV/LEV	54% (all) No significant difference	64% (all) No significant difference
INT 0144 (Smalley et al. 2003)[10]	2 cycles bolus 5-FU + RCT PVI 5-FU + 2 cycles bolus 5-FU PVI 5-FU + RCT PVI 5-FU + PVI 5-FU 2 cycles bolus 5-FU/LV/LEV + RCT bolus 5-FU/LV + 2 cycles bolus 5-FU/LV/LEV	68–69% (3years) No significant difference	81–83% (3 years) No significant difference
Korean Trial (Lee et al. 2002)[13]	RCT bolus FU/LV + 6 cycles bolus 5-FU/LV 2 cycles bolus 5-FU/LV + RCT bolus FU/LV + 4 cycles bolus 5-FU/LV	81% (4 years) 70% (4 years) $p = 0.04$	84% (4 years) 82% (4 years) $p = 0.39$

CT, chemotherapy; 5-FU, 5-fluorouracil; LEV, levamisol; LV, leucovorin; MeCCNU, 1-(2-chloroethyl)-3-(4-methylcyclohexyl)-1-nitrosourea; PVI, protracted venous infusion; RCT, radiochemotherapy; RT, radiotherapy.

downsizing effects that possibly enhance curative surgery in locally advanced disease, and sphincter preservation in low-lying tumours. The small bowel in an unviolated abdomen will be mobile and less likely to be within a pelvic radiation portal, the irradiated volume does not require coverage of the perineum, as in cases after abdominoperineal resection, and there is no irradiation of the anastomotic region. Thus, preoperative irradiation may cause less acute and late toxicity and more patients will receive full-dose therapy. In addition, a certain dose of irradiation seems to be more effective if given preoperatively compared with postoperatively, most probably due to the fact that oxygen tension within the tumour may be higher prior to surgical compromise of the regional blood flow. This may improve the radiosensitivity of the tumour by decreasing the more radioresistant hypoxic fraction.

Until recently the only randomized trial that directly compared preoperative to postoperative radiation therapy (both without chemotherapy) in rectal cancer has been the Uppsala trial, which was carried out between 1980 and 1985 in Sweden[14]. In the preoperative arm, patients received intensive short-course radiation (five fractions of 5.1 Gy to a total dose of 25.5 Gy in 1 week), postoperatively conventional radiation therapy (2 Gy to a total of 60 Gy with a 2-week split after 40 Gy) was applied. Preoperative radiation significantly decreased local failure rate (13% vs 22%, $p = 0.02$); however, there was no significant difference in 5-year survival rates (42% vs 38%).

Prospective randomized trials comparing the efficacy of preoperative radiochemotherapy to standard postoperative radiochemotherapy in UICC stage II and III rectal cancer were initiated both in the United States through the Radiation Therapy Oncology Group (RTOG 94-01) and the NSABP (R-03), as well as in Germany (Protocol CAO/ARO/AIO-94). Unfortunately, both US trials suffered from lack of accrual, and have already been closed. A preliminary report of the NSABP R-03 trial (with a median follow-up of only 1 year) revealed that the percentage of patients who underwent sphincter-sparing surgery and were without evidence of disease was higher in the preoperative versus the postoperative arm (44% vs 34%)[15].

The German multicentre study (CAO/ARO/AIO-94) has recently been completed, with more than 820 patients included. The design of this trial and the treatment schedule are depicted in Figure 1. Results were recently reported (Table 3)[16]: Compared with postoperative radiochemotherapy, the preoperative combined modality approach was superior in terms of local control, downstaging, acute and chronic toxicity, and sphincter preservation in those patients judged by the surgeon to require an abdominoperineal resection (APR). Given these advantages preoperative radiochemotherapy is now the preferred adjuvant treatment for patients with locally advanced rectal cancer in Germany, as well as in most parts of Europe. However, it needs to be emphasized that, with a median follow-up of 46 months, there was no difference in 5-year disease-free and overall survival rates between the two treatment arms.

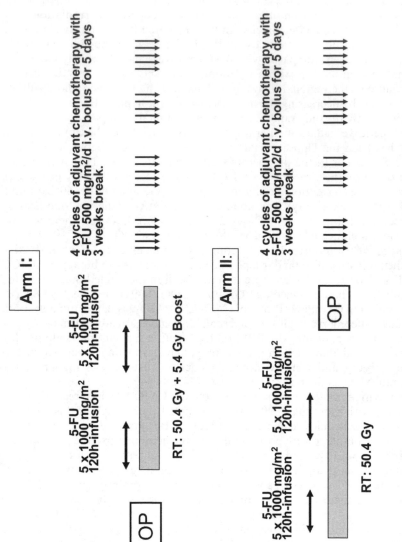

Figure 1 Design of the German CAO/ARO/AIO-94 study comparing postoperative (arm I) with preoperative radiochemotherapy (arm II) in locally advanced rectal cancer

Table 3 German Rectal Cancer Study Group randomized trial of preoperative compared with postoperative radiochemotherapy for rectal cancer[16]

5-year outcome	Preoperative RCT (%)	Postoperative RCT (%)	p-Value
Locoregional recurrence rate	6	13	0.006
Distant recurrence rate	36	38	0.84
Disease-free survival	68	65	0.32
Overall survival	74	76	0.80
Any grade 3/4-acute toxicity	27	40	0.001
Any grade 3/4-late toxicity	14	24	0.01
Sphincter preservation rate[a]	39	19	0.004

[a]In patients deemed to require abdominal–perineal resection by the surgeon before randomization.

DO WE NEED CONCOMITANT CHEMOTHERAPY WITH PREOPERATIVE RADIATION THERAPY?

The concurrent use of chemotherapy as part of the preoperative regimen is another important point, as it is not clear at present whether data from postoperative radiochemotherapy in resectable rectal cancer can be translated to the preoperative setting. For the treatment of primarily 'unresectable', fixed T4 rectal cancer, several institutions have applied preoperative radiation in conventional fractionation. The goal is to convert ('downsize') a tumour, which is clinically not amenable to curative resection at presentation, to a resectable status. Minsky et al. compared preoperative radiotherapy (50.4 Gy) with or without 5-FU/high-dose folinic acid and showed that 90% of the patients with initially 'unresectable' tumours were converted to resectable lesions by preoperative combined therapy as compared with only 64% of those who received radiation therapy alone[17]. Moreover, a complete pathological response was found in 20% of patients receiving combined-modality therapy as compared to 6% receiving radiotherapy alone, indicating an enhancement of radiation-induced 'downstaging' by concomitant 5-FU-based chemotherapy.

In a recent randomized phase III study comparing radiotherapy alone with combined radiochemotherapy for primarily unresectable rectal cancer, Frykholm et al. could demonstrate that the addition of chemotherapy to radiotherapy significantly improved local control rates, albeit again no significant difference in survival was found between the groups[18]. A Polish randomized trial compared preoperative short-course irradiation (5×5 Gy) and immediate surgery with conventionally fractionated radiochemotherapy (1.8 Gy to 50.4 Gy) and delayed surgery in 316 patients with locally advanced (T3/T4) low rectal cancer[19]. The primary endpoint of the trial was the rate of sphincter-preserving surgery. Despite a significant increase in tumour response in the radiochemotherapy group (pathological complete remission, 16% vs 1%; mean largest tumour diameter on the operative specimen, 29 mm vs 48 mm), the rate of sphincter preservation was 61% in the immediate surgery group and 58% in the delayed group, indicating a strong commitment of the surgeons in this trial not to change their choice whatever the tumour response was after neoadjuvant radiochemotherapy.

Table 4 Preoperative conventionally fractionated radiotherapy with or without 5-FU/LV-based chemotherapy. Results of EORTC 22921 and FFCD 9203 randomized trials[20,21]

5-year outcome	Preoperative RT	Preoperative RCT	p-Value
EORTC 22921 (n = 1011)			
pCR rate	5.3%	13.7%	<0.001
ypN0	60.5%	71.9%	<0.001
Tumour size (median)	30 mm	25 mm	<0.0001
Sphincter preserved	52.4%	55.6%	0.05
Local failure	17%	8%	0.002
Overall survival	64.8%	65.6%	0.79
FFCD 9203 (n = 762)			
pCR rate	3.7%	11.7%	<0.0001
Sphincter preserved	52.6%	51.7%	n.s.
Grade 3+4 toxicity	2.7%	14.6%	<0.0001
Local failure	8%	16.5%	n.g.
Overall survival	66%	67%	n.g.

n.s., not significant; n.g., not given.

In primarily respectable tumours (cT3/4 and/or cN+), the European Organization for Research and Treatment of Cancer (EORTC study 22921) has conducted a four-arm trial that treated all patients with preoperative radiation in conventional fractionation (45 Gy in 25 fractions) and tested whether preoperative concurrent radiochemotherapy with 5-FU/leucovorin, postoperative 5-FU/leucovorin, or both are superior to preoperative radiation alone (Table 4)[20]. The FFCD 9203 was a two-arm trial also randomizing patients to preoperative 45 Gy with or without bolus 5-FU/leucovorin[21]. All patients received postoperative chemotherapy in this trial. First results of both trails were reported at ASCO 2005 and indicated that the addition of 5-FU/leucovorin to preoperative conventionally fractionated radiation therapy significantly increased the pathological complete response rates, reduced tumour size and lymph nodal invasion, increased sphincter preservation (in EORTC 22921 only) and long-term local control rates; yet these advantages once again did not translate into a survival benefit for patients treated by combined radiation and chemotherapy.

INTEGRATING NOVEL CHEMOTHERAPEUTIC AGENTS INTO PREOPERATIVE COMBINED MODALITY TREATMENT FOR RECTAL CANCER

Given that – with optimized local treatment, including preoperative radiotherapy and TME (total mesorectal excision) surgery – distant metastasis is by far the predominant pattern of tumour failure in rectal cancer today, the future challenge is to integrate more effective systemic therapy into the multimodal concepts for this disease. Novel chemotherapeutic agents such as capecitabine, oxaliplatin, and irinotecan, as well as targeted therapies, such as bevacizumab and cetuximab, which have improved results of patients treated

Table 5 Selected phase II studies of preoperative chemoradiotherapy for locally advanced rectal cancer using oxaliplatin-based combined-modality treatment

Series	n	Concurrent chemoradiotherapy	Toxicity	pCR*
Carraro et al. 2002[23]	22	Preop. RT: 1.8 Gy to 50.4 Gy. Days 1–4 and 29–32: 5-FU 375 mg/m² per day, LV 20 mg/m² per day, oxaliplatin 25 mg/m² per day; day 15: oxaliplatin 50 mg/m². Four weeks after RT, one additional cycle of oxaliplatin, 5-FU/LV (same dose as during RT)	Grade 4: leucopenia 4.5%. Grade 3: diarrhoea 27%, leukopenia 4.5%	25%
Gérard et al. 2003[24]	40	Preop. RT: 1.8 Gy to 45 Gy (concomitant boost to 50 Gy). Days 1–5 and 29–33: 5-FU 350 mg/m² per day, LV 100 mg/m² per day; days 1 and 29: oxaliplatin 130 mg/m² per day	Grade 4: diarrhea 2.5%, mucositis 2.5%. Grade 3: fatigue 7.5%, diarrhoea 5%, proctitis 5%, neutropenia 2.5%	15%
Rödel et al. 2003[25]	26	Preop. RT: 1.8 Gy to 50.4 Gy. Days 1–14 and 22–35: capecitabine 825 mg/m² b.i.d.; days 1, 8 and 22, 29: oxaliplatin 50 mg/m² per day	Grade 3: diarrhoea 8%, skin (local) 8%	19%
Gambacorta et al. 2004[26]	30	Preop. RT: 1.8 Gy to 50.4 Gy. Days 1, 19, 38: Raltitrexed 3 mg/m² per day, oxaliplatin 130 mg/m² per day	Grade 3: leucopenia 10%, vomiting 3%, proctitis 3%	30%
Aschele et al. 2005[27]	25	Preop. RT: 1.8 Gy to 50.4 Gy. Duration of RT: 5-FU 225 mg/m² per day, oxaliplatin 60 mg/m² per day once weekly for a total of 6 courses.	Grade 3: diarrhoea 15%, skin (local) 12%, anaemia 4%	28%

5-FU, 5-fluorouracil; LV, leucovorin; pCR, pathological complete response; RT, radiotherapy.

175

Table 6 Selected phase II studies of preoperative chemoradiotherapy for locally advanced rectal cancer using irinotecan-based combined-modality treatment

Series	n	Concurrent chemoradiotherapy	Toxicity	pCR*
Mehta et al. 2003[28]	32	Preop. RT: 1.8 Gy to 50.4 Gy Days 1–33: 5-FU 200 mg/m² per day; days 1, 8, 15, 22: CPT-11 50 mg/m² per day	Grade 3: diarrhoea 28%, mucositis 21%, proctitis 21%, abdominal cramping 9%	37%
Klautke et al. 2005[29]	37	Preop. RT: 1.8 Gy to 50.4 Gy Duration of RT: 5-FU 250 mg/m² per day; CPT-11 40 mg/m² per day once weekly for a total of 6 courses	Grade 4: diarrhoea 5%, leucopenia 2% Grade 3: diarrhoea 27%, leucopenia 8%	22%

CPT-II, trinotecan; pCR, pathological complete response.

in the adjuvant and metastatic setting for colorectal cancer, are currently incorporated into phase I/II combined modality programmes for rectal cancer as well (Tables 5 and 6). All suggest higher pathological complete response (pCR) rates compared with 5-FU-radiochemotherapy alone. However, for some agents, with this increased pCR rate comes an associated increase in acute toxicity. Clearly, phase III trials are needed to determine if these regimens offer an advantage compared with a 5-FU-based combined-modality regimen.

References

1. Gastrointestinal Tumor Study Group: Prolongation of the disease-free interval in surgically treated rectal carcinoma. N Engl J Med. 1985;312:1465–72.
2. Krook JE, Moertel CG, Gunderson LL et al. Effective surgical adjuvant therapy for high risk rectal carcinoma. N Engl J Med. 1991;324:709–15.
3. Tveit KM, Guldvog I, Hagen S et al. Randomized controlled trial of postoperative radiotherapy and short-term time-scheduled 5-fluorouracil against surgery alone in the treatment of Dukes B and C rectal cancer. Norwegian Adjuvant Rectal Cancer Project Group. Br J Surg. 1997;84:1130–5.
4. Fisher B, Wolmark N, Rockette H et al. Postoperative adjuvant chemotherapy or radiation therapy for rectal cancer: results from NSABP protocol R-01. J Natl Cancer Inst. 1988;80:21–9.
5. Wolmark N, Wieand HS, Hyams DM et al. Randomized trial of postoperative adjuvant chemotherapy with or without radiotherapy for carcinoma of the rectum: National Surgical Adjuvant Breast and Bowel Project Protocol R-02. J Natl Cancer Inst. 2000;92:388–96.
6. Cafiero F, Gipponi M, Lionetto R. Randomised clinical trial of adjuvant postoperative RT vs. sequential postoperative RT plus 5-FU and levamisole in patients with stage II-III resectable rectal cancer: a final report. J Surg Oncol. 2003;83:140–6.
7. NIH Consensus Conference. Adjuvant therapy for patients with colon and rectal cancer. J Am Med Assoc. 1990;264:1444–50.
8. Gastrointestinal Tumor Study Group: Radiation therapy and fluorouracil with or without semustine for the treatment of patients with surgical adjuvant adenocarcinoma of the rectum. J Clin Oncol. 1992;10:549–57.
9. O'Connell MJ, Martenson JA, Wieand HS et al. Improving adjuvant therapy for rectal cancer by combining protracted-infusion fluorouracil with radiation therapy after curative surgery. N Engl J Med. 1994;331:502–7.
10. Smalley SR, Benedetti J, Williamson S et al. Intergroup 0144 – phase III trial of 5-FU based chemotherapy regimens plus radiotherapy (XRT) in postoperative adjuvant rectal cancer. Bolus 5-FU vs prolonged venous infusion (PVI) before and after XRT + PVI vs bolus 5-FU + leucovorin (LV) + levamisole (LEV) before and after XRT + bolus 5-FU + LV. Proc Am Soc Clin Oncol. 2003; Abstract 1006.
11. Tepper JE, O'Connell M, Niedzwiecki D et al. Adjuvant therapy in rectal cancer: analysis of stage, sex, and local control – final report of intergroup 0114. J Clin Oncol. 2002;20:1744–50.
12. Staib L, Kornmann M, Roettinger E et al. Adjuvant radiochemotherapy in resectable stage II, III rectal cancer: results of the FOGT-2 trial. Proc Am Soc Clin Oncol. 2004; Abstract 3608.
13. Lee JH, Ahn JH, Bahng H et al. Randomized trial of postoperative adjuvant therapy in stage II and III rectal cancer to define the optimal sequence of chemotherapy and radiotherapy: a preliminary report. J Clin Oncol. 2002;20:1751–8.
14. Frykholm GJ, Glimelius B, Pahlman L. Preoperative or postoperative irradiation in adenocarcinoma of the rectum: final treatment results of a randomized trial and an evaluation of late secondary effects. Dis Colon Rectum. 1993;36:564–72.
15. Roh MS, Petrelli N, Wieand S et al. Phase III randomized trial of preoperative versus postoperative multimodality therapy in patients with carcinoma of the rectum (NSABP R-03). Proc Am Soc Clin Oncol. 2001;20:123a.
16. Sauer R, Becker H, Hohenberger W et al. Preoperative versus postoperative chemoradiotherapy for rectal cancer. N Engl J Med. 2004;351:1731–40.

17. Minsky BD, Cohen AM, Kemeny N et al. Enhancement of radiation-induced downstaging of rectal cancer by fluorouracil and high-dose leucovorin chemotherapy. J Clin Oncol. 1992;10:79–84.
18. Frykholm GJ, Påhlman L, Glimelius B. Combined chemo- and radiotherapy vs. radiotherapy alone in the treatment of primary, nonresectable adenocarcinoma of the rectum. Int J Radiat Oncol Biol Phys. 2001;50:427–34.
19. Bujko K, Nowacki MP, Nasierowska-Guttmejer A et al. Sphincter preservation following preoperative radiotherapy for rectal cancer: report of a randomised trial comparing short-term radiotherapy vs. conventionally fractionated radiochemotherapy. Radiother Oncol. 2004;72:15–24.
20. Bosset JF, Calais G, Mineur L et al. Preoperative radiation (Preop RT) in rectal cancer: effect and timing of additional chemotherapy (CT) 5-year results of the EORTC 22921 trial. Proc Am Soc Clin Oncol. 2005; Abstract 3505.
21. Gerard JP, Bonnetain F, Conroy T et al. Preoperative (preop) radiotherapy (RT) + 5 FU/folinic acid (FA) in T3-4 rectal cancers: results of the FFCD 9203 randomized trial. Proc Am Soc Clin Oncol. 2005; Abstract 3504.
22. Fountzilas G, Zisiadis A, Dafni U et al: Postoperative radiation and concomitant bolus fluorouracil with or without additional chemotherapy with fluorouracil and high-dose leucovorin in patients with high-risk rectal cancer: a randomized phase III study conducted by the Hellenic Cooperative Oncology Group. Ann Oncol. 1999;10:671–6.
23. Carraro S, Roca EL, Cartelli C et al. Radiochemotherapy with short daily infusion of low-dose oxaliplatin, leucovorin, and 5-FU in T3-T4 unresectable rectal cancer: a phase II IATTGI study. Int J Radiat Oncol Biol Phys. 2002;54:397–402.
24. Gerard JP, Chapet O, Nemoz C et al. Preoperative concurrent chemoradiotherapy in locally advanced rectal cancer with high-dose radiation and oxaliplatin-containing regimen: the Lyon R0-04 phase II trial. J Clin Oncol. 2003;21:1119–24.
25. Rödel C, Grabenbauer GG, Papadopoulos T et al. Phase I/II trial of capecitabine, oxaliplatin, and radiation for rectal cancer. J Clin Oncol. 2003;21:3098–104.
26. Gambacorta MA, Valentini V, Coco C et al. Chemoradiation with raltitrexed and oxaliplatin in preoperative treatment of stage II-III resectable rectal cancer: Phase I and II studies. Int J Radiat Oncol Biol Phys. 2004;60:139–48.
27. Aschele C, Friso ML, Pucciarelli S et al. A phase I-II study of weekly oxaliplatin, 5-fluorouracil continuous infusion and preoperative radiotherapy in locally advanced rectal cancer. Ann Oncol. 2005;16:1140–6.
28. Mehta VK, Cho C, Ford JM et al. Phase II trial of preoperative 3D conformal radiotherapy, protracted venous infusion 5-fluorouracil, and weekly CPT-11, followed by surgery for ultrasound-staged T3 rectal cancer. Int J Radiat Oncol Biol Phys. 2003;55:132–7.
29. Klautke G, Feyerherd P, Ludwig K et al. Intensified concurrent chemoradiotherapy with 5-fluorouracil and irinotecan as neoadjuvant treatment in patients with locally advanced rectal cancer. Br J Cancer. 2005;92:1215–20.

Index

Falk Symposium Series

43. Reutter W, Popper H, Arias IM, Heinrich PC, Keppler D, Landmann L, eds.: *Modulation of Liver Cell Expression*. Falk Symposium No. 43. 1987
ISBN: 0-85200-677-2*
44. Boyer JL, Bianchi L, eds.: *Liver Cirrhosis*. Falk Symposium No. 44. 1987
ISBN: 0-85200-993-3*
45. Paumgartner G, Stiehl A, Gerok W, eds.: *Bile Acids and the Liver*. Falk Symposium No. 45. 1987
ISBN: 0-85200-675-6*
46. Goebell H, Peskar BM, Malchow H, eds.: *Inflammatory Bowel Diseases – Basic Research & Clinical Implications*. Falk Symposium No. 46. 1988
ISBN: 0-7462-0067-6*
47. Bianchi L, Holt P, James OFW, Butler RN, eds.: *Aging in Liver and Gastrointestinal Tract*. Falk Symposium No. 47. 1988
ISBN: 0-7462-0066-8*
48. Heilmann C, ed.: *Calcium-Dependent Processes in the Liver*. Falk Symposium No. 48. 1988
ISBN: 0-7462-0075-7*
50. Singer MV, Goebell H, eds.: *Nerves and the Gastrointestinal Tract*. Falk Symposium No. 50. 1989
ISBN: 0-7462-0114-1
51. Bannasch P, Keppler D, Weber G, eds.: *Liver Cell Carcinoma*. Falk Symposium No. 51. 1989
ISBN: 0-7462-0111-7
52. Paumgartner G, Stiehl A, Gerok W, eds.: *Trends in Bile Acid Research*. Falk Symposium No. 52. 1989
ISBN: 0-7462-0112-5
53. Paumgartner G, Stiehl A, Barbara L, Roda E, eds.: *Strategies for the Treatment of Hepatobiliary Diseases*. Falk Symposium No. 53. 1990 ISBN: 0-7923-8903-4
54. Bianchi L, Gerok W, Maier K-P, Deinhardt F, eds.: *Infectious Diseases of the Liver*. Falk Symposium No. 54. 1990
ISBN: 0-7923-8902-6
55. Falk Symposium No. 55 not published
55B. Hadziselimovic F, Herzog B, Bürgin-Wolff A, eds.: *Inflammatory Bowel Disease and Coeliac Disease in Children*. International Falk Symposium. 1990
ISBN 0-7462-0125-7
56. Williams CN, eds.: *Trends in Inflammatory Bowel Disease Therapy*. Falk Symposium No. 56. 1990
ISBN: 0-7923-8952-2
57. Bock KW, Gerok W, Matern S, Schmid R, eds.: *Hepatic Metabolism and Disposition of Endo- and Xenobiotics*. Falk Symposium No. 57. 1991 ISBN: 0-7923-8953-0
58. Paumgartner G, Stiehl A, Gerok W, eds.: *Bile Acids as Therapeutic Agents: From Basic Science to Clinical Practice*. Falk Symposium No. 58. 1991 ISBN: 0-7923-8954-9
59. Halter F, Garner A, Tytgat GNJ, eds.: *Mechanisms of Peptic Ulcer Healing*. Falk Symposium No. 59. 1991
ISBN: 0-7923-8955-7
60. Goebell H, Ewe K, Malchow H, Koelbel Ch, eds.: *Inflammatory Bowel Diseases – Progress in Basic Research and Clinical Implications*. Falk Symposium No. 60. 1991
ISBN: 0-7923-8956-5
61. Falk Symposium No. 61 not published
62. Dowling RH, Folsch UR, Löser Ch, eds.: *Polyamines in the Gastrointestinal Tract*. Falk Symposium No. 62. 1992
ISBN: 0-7923-8976-X
63. Lentze MJ, Reichen J, eds.: *Paediatric Cholestasis: Novel Approaches to Treatment*. Falk Symposium No. 63. 1992
ISBN: 0-7923-8977-8
64. Demling L, Frühmorgen P, eds.: *Non-Neoplastic Diseases of the Anorectum*. Falk Symposium No. 64. 1992
ISBN: 0-7923-8979-4
64B. Gressner AM, Ramadori G, eds.: *Molecular and Cell Biology of Liver Fibrogenesis*. International Falk Symposium. 1992
ISBN: 0-7923-8980-8

*These titles were published under the MTP Press imprint.

Falk Symposium Series

65. Hadziselimovic F, Herzog B, eds.: *Inflammatory Bowel Diseases and Morbus Hirschprung*. Falk Symposium No. 65. 1992   ISBN: 0-7923-8995-6
66. Martin F, McLeod RS, Sutherland LR, Williams CN, eds.: *Trends in Inflammatory Bowel Disease Therapy*. Falk Symposium No. 66. 1993   ISBN: 0-7923-8827-5
67. Schölmerich J, Kruis W, Goebell H, Hohenberger W, Gross V, eds.: *Inflammatory Bowel Diseases – Pathophysiology as Basis of Treatment*. Falk Symposium No. 67. 1993
          ISBN: 0-7923-8996-4
68. Paumgartner G, Stiehl A, Gerok W, eds.: *Bile Acids and The Hepatobiliary System: From Basic Science to Clinical Practice*. Falk Symposium No. 68. 1993
          ISBN: 0-7923-8829-1
69. Schmid R, Bianchi L, Gerok W, Maier K-P, eds.: *Extrahepatic Manifestations in Liver Diseases*. Falk Symposium No. 69. 1993   ISBN: 0-7923-8821-6
70. Meyer zum Büschenfelde K-H, Hoofnagle J, Manns M, eds.: *Immunology and Liver*. Falk Symposium No. 70. 1993   ISBN: 0-7923-8830-5
71. Surrenti C, Casini A, Milani S, Pinzani M , eds.: *Fat-Storing Cells and Liver Fibrosis*. Falk Symposium No. 71. 1994   ISBN: 0-7923-8842-9
72. Rachmilewitz D, ed.: *Inflammatory Bowel Diseases – 1994*. Falk Symposium No. 72. 1994   ISBN: 0-7923-8845-3
73. Binder HJ, Cummings J, Soergel KH, eds.: *Short Chain Fatty Acids*. Falk Symposium No. 73. 1994   ISBN: 0-7923-8849-6
73B. Möllmann HW, May B, eds.: *Glucocorticoid Therapy in Chronic Inflammatory Bowel Disease: from basic principles to rational therapy*. International Falk Workshop. 1996
          ISBN 0-7923-8708-2
74. Keppler D, Jungermann K, eds.: *Transport in the Liver*. Falk Symposium No. 74. 1994
          ISBN: 0-7923-8858-5
74B. Stange EF, ed.: *Chronic Inflammatory Bowel Disease*. Falk Symposium. 1995
          ISBN: 0-7923-8876-3
75. van Berge Henegouwen GP, van Hoek B, De Groote J, Matern S, Stockbrügger RW, eds.: *Cholestatic Liver Diseases: New Strategies for Prevention and Treatment of Hepatobiliary and Cholestatic Liver Diseases*. Falk Symposium 75. 1994.
          ISBN: 0-7923-8867-4
76. Monteiro E, Tavarela Veloso F, eds.: *Inflammatory Bowel Diseases: New Insights into Mechanisms of Inflammation and Challenges in Diagnosis and Treatment*. Falk Symposium 76. 1995.   ISBN 0-7923-8884-4
77. Singer MV, Ziegler R, Rohr G, eds.: *Gastrointestinal Tract and Endocrine System*. Falk Symposium 77. 1995.   ISBN 0-7923-8877-1
78. Decker K, Gerok W, Andus T, Gross V, eds.: *Cytokines and the Liver*. Falk Symposium 78. 1995.   ISBN 0-7923-8878-X
79. Holstege A, Schölmerich J, Hahn EG, eds.: *Portal Hypertension*. Falk Symposium 79. 1995.   ISBN 0-7923-8879-8
80. Hofmann AF, Paumgartner G, Stiehl A, eds.: *Bile Acids in Gastroenterology: Basic and Clinical Aspects*. Falk Symposium 80. 1995   ISBN 0-7923-8880-1
81. Riecken EO, Stallmach A, Zeitz M, Heise W, eds.: *Malignancy and Chronic Inflammation in the Gastrointestinal Tract – New Concepts*. Falk Symposium 81. 1995
ISBN 0-7923-8889-5
82. Fleig WE, ed.: *Inflammatory Bowel Diseases: New Developments and Standards*. Falk Symposium 82. 1995   ISBN 0-7923-8890-6

Falk Symposium Series

Falk Symposium Series

Falk Symposium Series

116A. Dienes HP, Schirmacher P, Brechot C, Okuda K, eds. *Chronic Hepatitis: New Concepts of Pathogenesis, Diagnosis and Treatment.* Falk Workshop. 2000
ISBN 0-7923-8763-5

117. Gerbes AL, Beuers U, Jüngst D, Pape GR, Sackmann M, Sauerbruch T, eds. *Hepatology 2000 – Symposium in Honour of Gustav Paumgartner.* Falk Symposium 117. 2000
ISBN 0-7923-8765-1

117A. Acalovschi M, Paumgartner G, eds. *Hepatobiliary Diseases: Cholestasis and Gallstones.* Falk Workshop. 2000
ISBN 0-7923-8770-8

118. Frühmorgen P, Bruch H-P, eds. *Non-Neoplastic Diseases of the Anorectum.* Falk Symposium 118. 2001
ISBN 0-7923-8766-X

119. Fellermann K, Jewell DP, Sandborn WJ, Schölmerich J, Stange EF, eds. *Immunosuppression in Inflammatory Bowel Diseases – Standards, New Developments, Future Trends.* Falk Symposium 119. 2001
ISBN 0-7923-8767-8

120. van Berge Henegouwen GP, Keppler D, Leuschner U, Paumgartner G, Stiehl A, eds. *Biology of Bile Acids in Health and Disease.* Falk Symposium 120. 2001
ISBN 0-7923-8768-6

121. Leuschner U, James OFW, Dancygier H, eds. *Steatohepatitis (NASH and ASH).* Falk Symposium 121. 2001
ISBN 0-7923-8769-4

121A. Matern S, Boyer JL, Keppler D, Meier-Abt PJ, eds. *Hepatobiliary Transport: From Bench to Bedside.* Falk Workshop. 2001
ISBN 0-7923-8771-6

122. Campieri M, Fiocchi C, Hanauer SB, Jewell DP, Rachmilewitz R, Schölmerich J, eds. *Inflammatory Bowel Disease – A Clinical Case Approach to Pathophysiology, Diagnosis, and Treatment.* Falk Symposium 122. 2002
ISBN 0-7923-8772-4

123. Rachmilewitz D, Modigliani R, Podolsky DK, Sachar DB, Tozun N, eds. *VI International Symposium on Inflammatory Bowel Diseases.* Falk Symposium 123. 2002
ISBN 0-7923-8773-2

124. Hagenmüller F, Manns MP, Musmann H-G, Riemann JF, eds. *Medical Imaging in Gastroenterology and Hepatology.* Falk Symposium 124. 2002 ISBN 0-7923-8774-0

125. Gressner AM, Heinrich PC, Matern S, eds. *Cytokines in Liver Injury and Repair.* Falk Symposium 125. 2002
ISBN 0-7923-8775-9

126. Gupta S, Jansen PLM, Klempnauer J, Manns MP, eds. *Hepatocyte Transplantation.* Falk Symposium 126. 2002
ISBN 0-7923-8776-7

127. Hadziselimovic F, ed. *Autoimmune Diseases in Paediatric Gastroenterology.* Falk Symposium 127. 2002
ISBN 0-7923-8778-3

127A. Berr F, Bruix J, Hauss J, Wands J, Wittekind Ch, eds. *Malignant Liver Tumours: Basic Concepts and Clinical Management.* Falk Workshop. 2002
ISBN 0-7923-8779-1

128. Scheppach W, Scheurlen M, eds. *Exogenous Factors in Colonic Carcinogenesis.* Falk Symposium 128. 2002
ISBN 0-7923-8780-5

129. Paumgartner G, Keppler D, Leuschner U, Stiehl A, eds. *Bile Acids: From Genomics to Disease and Therapy.* Falk Symposium 129. 2002
ISBN 0-7923-8781-3

129A. Leuschner U, Berg PA, Holtmeier J, eds. *Bile Acids and Pregnancy.* Falk Workshop. 2002
ISBN 0-7923-8782-1

130. Holtmann G, Talley NJ, eds. *Gastrointestinal Inflammation and Disturbed Gut Function: The Challenge of New Concepts.* Falk Symposium 130. 2003
ISBN 0-7923-8783-X

131. Herfarth H, Feagan BJ, Folsch UR, Schölmerich J, Vatn MH, Zeitz M, eds. *Targets of Treatment in Chronic Inflammatory Bowel Diseases.* Falk Symposium 131. 2003
ISBN 0-7923-8784-8

Falk Symposium Series

132. Galle PR, Gerken G, Schmidt WE, Wiedenmann B, eds. *Disease Progression and Carcinogenesis in the Gastrointestinal Tract*. Falk Symposium 132. 2003
ISBN 0-7923-8785-6
132A. Staritz M, Adler G, Knuth A, Schmiegel W, Schmoll H-J, eds. *Side-effects of Chemotherapy on the Gastrointestinal Tract*. Falk Workshop. 2003
ISBN 0-7923-8791-0
132B. Reutter W, Schuppan D, Tauber R, Zeitz M, eds. *Cell Adhesion Molecules in Health and Disease*. Falk Workshop. 2003   ISBN 0-7923-8786-4
133. Duchmann R, Blumberg R, Neurath M, Schölmerich J, Strober W, Zeitz M. *Mechanisms of Intestinal Inflammation: Implications for Therapeutic Intervention in IBD*. Falk Symposium 133. 2004   ISBN 0-7923-8787-2
134. Dignass A, Lochs H, Stange E. *Trends and Controversies in IBD – Evidence-Based Approach or Individual Management?* Falk Symposium 134. 2004
ISBN 0-7923-8788-0
134A. Dignass A, Gross HJ, Buhr V, James OFW. *Topical Steroids in Gastroenterology and Hepatology*. Falk Workshop. 2004   ISBN 0-7923-8789-9
135. Lukáš M, Manns MP, Špičák J, Stange EF, eds. *Immunological Diseases of Liver and Gut*. Falk Symposium 135. 2004   ISBN 0-7923-8792-9
136. Leuschner U, Broomé U, Stiehl A, eds. *Cholestatic Liver Diseases: Therapeutic Options and Perspectives*. Falk Symposium 136. 2004   ISBN 0-7923-8793-7
137. Blum HE, Maier KP, Rodés J, Sauerbruch T, eds. *Liver Diseases: Advances in Treatment and Prevention*. Falk Symposium 137. 2004   ISBN 0-7923-8794-5
138. Blum HE, Manns MP, eds. *State of the Art of Hepatology: Molecular and Cell Biology*. Falk Symposium 138. 2004   ISBN 0-7923-8795-3
138A. Hayashi N, Manns MP, eds. *Prevention of Progression in Chronic Liver Disease: An Update on SNMC (Stronger Neo-Minophagen C)*. Falk Workshop. 2004
ISBN 0-7923-8796-1
139. Adler G, Blum HE, Fuchs M, Stange EF, eds. *Gallstones: Pathogenesis and Treatment*. Falk Symposium 139. 2004   ISBN 0-7923-8798-8
140. Colombel J-F, Gasché C, Schölmerich J, Vucelic C, eds. *Inflammatory Bowel Disease: Translation from Basic Research to Clinical Practice*. Falk Symposium 140. 2005.   ISBN 1-4020-2847-4
141. Paumgartner G, Keppler D, Leuschner U, Stiehl A, eds. *Bile Acid Biology and its Therapeutic Implications*. Falk Symposium 141. 2005   ISBN 1-4020-2893-8
142. Dienes H-P, Leuschner U, Lohse AW, Manns MP, eds. *Autoimmune Liver Disease*. Falk Symposium 142. 2005   ISBN 1-4020-2894-6
143. Ammann RW, Büchler MW, Adler G, DiMagno EP, Sarner M, eds. *Pancreatitis: Advances in Pathobiology, Diagnosis and Treatment*. Falk Symposium 143. 2005
ISBN 1-4020-2895-4
144. Adler G, Blum AL, Blum HE, Leuschner U, Manns MP, Mössner J, Sartor RB, Schölmerich J, eds. *Gastroenterology Yesterday – Today – Tomorrow: A Review and Preview*. Falk Symposium 144. 2005   ISBN 1-4020-2896-2
145. Henne-Bruns D, Buttenschön K, Fuchs M, Lohse AW, eds. *Artificial Liver Support*. Falk Symposium 145. 2005   ISBN 1-4020-3239-0
146. Blumberg RS, Gangl A, Manns MP, Tilg H, Zeitz M, eds. *Gut–Liver Interactions: Basic and Clinical Concepts*. Falk Symposium 146. 2005   ISBN 1-4020-4143-8
147. Jewell DP, Colombel JF, Peña AS, Tromm A, Warren BS, eds. *Colitis: Diagnosis and Therapeutic Strategies*. Falk Symposium 147. 2006   ISBN 1-4020-4315-5

Falk Symposium Series

148. Kruis W, Forbes A, Jauch K-W, Kreis ME, Wexner SD, eds. *Diverticular Disease: Emerging Evidence in a Common Condition.* Falk Symposium 148. 2006
ISBN 1-4020- 4317-1

149. van Cutsem E, Rustgi AK., Schmiegel W, Zeitz M, eds. *Highlights in Gastrointestinal Oncology.* Falk Symposium 149. 2006.   ISBN 1-4020-5108-5

150. Galle PR, Gerken G, Schmidt WE, Wiedenmann B, eds. *Disease Progression and Disease Prevention in Hepatology and Gastroenterology.* Falk Symposium 150. 2006
ISBN 1-4020-5109-3